50% OFF
Online NHA Phlebotomy Prep Course!

By Mometrix

Dear Customer,

We consider it an honor and a privilege that you chose our NHA Phlebotomy Study Guide. As a way of showing our appreciation and to help us better serve you, we are offering **50% off our online NHA Phlebotomy Prep Course**. Many NHA Phlebotomy courses are needlessly expensive and don't deliver enough value. With our course, you get access to the best NHA Phlebotomy prep material, and **you only pay half price**.

We have structured our online course to perfectly complement your printed study guide. The NHA Phlebotomy Prep Course contains **in-depth lessons** that cover all the most important topics, over **800 practice questions** to ensure you feel prepared, and more than **300 digital flashcards**, so you can study while you're on the go.

Online NHA Phlebotomy Prep Course

Topics Included:

- Safety and Compliance
  - Legal and Professional Considerations
  - Laboratory Infection Control
- Patient Preparation
  - Laboratory Orders
  - Medical Terminology
- Routine Blood Collections
  - Specific Blood Tests
  - Point of Care Tests
- Special Collections
- Processing

Course Features:

- NHA Phlebotomy Study Guide
  - Get content that complements our best-selling study guide.
- Full-Length Practice Tests
  - With over 800 practice questions, you can test yourself again and again.
- Mobile Friendly
  - If you need to study on the go, the course is easily accessible from your mobile device.
- NHA Phlebotomy Flashcards
  - Our course includes a flashcard mode with over 300 content cards to help you study.

To receive this discount, visit us at mometrix.com/university/nha-phlebotomy or simply scan this QR code with your smartphone. At the checkout page, enter the discount code: **nha50off**

If you have any questions or concerns, please contact us at support@mometrix.com.

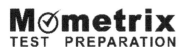

FREE Study Skills Videos/DVD Offer

Dear Customer,

Thank you for your purchase from Mometrix! We consider it an honor and a privilege that you have purchased our product and we want to ensure your satisfaction.

As part of our ongoing effort to meet the needs of test takers, we have developed a set of Study Skills Videos that we would like to give you for <u>FREE</u>. These videos cover our *best practices* for getting ready for your exam, from how to use our study materials to how to best prepare for the day of the test.

All that we ask is that you email us with feedback that would describe your experience so far with our product. Good, bad, or indifferent, we want to know what you think!

To get your FREE Study Skills Videos, you can use the **QR code** below, or send us an **email** at <u>studyvideos@mometrix.com</u> with *FREE VIDEOS* in the subject line and the following information in the body of the email:

- The name of the product you purchased.
- Your product rating on a scale of 1-5, with 5 being the highest rating.
- Your feedback. It can be long, short, or anything in between. We just want to know your impressions and experience so far with our product. (Good feedback might include how our study material met your needs and ways we might be able to make it even better. You could highlight features that you found helpful or features that you think we should add.)

If you have any questions or concerns, please don't hesitate to contact me directly.

Thanks again!

Sincerely,

Jay Willis
Vice President
<u>jay.willis@mometrix.com</u>
1-800-673-8175

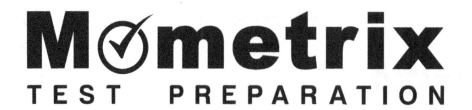

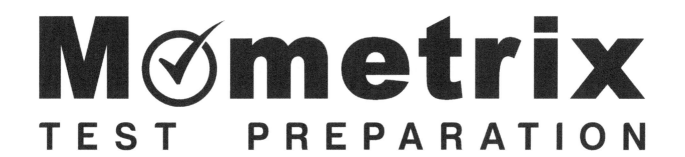

NHA Phlebotomy

Study Guide 2025-2026

4 Full-Length Practice Tests

Secrets Exam Prep Book for the NHA Certification

5th Edition

NHA Phlebotomy Study Guide - Full-Length Practice Tests, Secrets Exam Prep Book for the NHA Certification: [5th Edition]

Written and edited by Matthew Bowling

Printed in the United States of America

This paper meets the requirements of ANSI/NISO Z39.48-1992 (Permanence of Paper).

Mometrix offers volume discount pricing to institutions. For more information or a price quote, please contact our sales department at sales@mometrix.com or 888-248-1219.

Mometrix Media LLC is not affiliated with or endorsed by any official testing organization. All organizational and test names are trademarks of their respective owners.

Paperback
ISBN 13: 978-1-5167-2706-3
ISBN 10: 1-5167-2706-1

DEAR FUTURE EXAM SUCCESS STORY

First of all, **THANK YOU** for purchasing Mometrix study materials!

Second, congratulations! You are one of the few determined test-takers who are committed to doing whatever it takes to excel on your exam. **You have come to the right place.** We developed these study materials with one goal in mind: to deliver you the information you need in a format that's concise and easy to use.

In addition to optimizing your guide for the content of the test, we've outlined our recommended steps for breaking down the preparation process into small, attainable goals so you can make sure you stay on track.

We've also analyzed the entire test-taking process, identifying the most common pitfalls and showing how you can overcome them and be ready for any curveball the test throws you.

Standardized testing is one of the biggest obstacles on your road to success, which only increases the importance of doing well in the high-pressure, high-stakes environment of test day. Your results on this test could have a significant impact on your future, and this guide provides the information and practical advice to help you achieve your full potential on test day.

Your success is our success

We would love to hear from you! If you would like to share the story of your exam success or if you have any questions or comments in regard to our products, please contact us at **800-673-8175** or **support@mometrix.com**.

Thanks again for your business and we wish you continued success!

Sincerely,
The Mometrix Test Preparation Team

Need more help? Check out our flashcards at:
http://MometrixFlashcards.com/Phlebotomy

---

ii

TABLE OF CONTENTS

Introduction

Thank you for purchasing this resource! You have made the choice to prepare yourself for a test that could have a huge impact on your future, and this guide is designed to help you be fully ready for test day. Obviously, it's important to have a solid understanding of the test material, but you also need to be prepared for the unique environment and stressors of the test, so that you can perform to the best of your abilities.

For this purpose, the first section that appears in this guide is the **Secret Keys**. We've devoted countless hours to meticulously researching what works and what doesn't, and we've boiled down our findings to the five most impactful steps you can take to improve your performance on the test. We start at the beginning with study planning and move through the preparation process, all the way to the testing strategies that will help you get the most out of what you know when you're finally sitting in front of the test.

We recommend that you start preparing for your test as far in advance as possible. However, if you've bought this guide as a last-minute study resource and only have a few days before your test, we recommend that you skip over the first two Secret Keys since they address a long-term study plan.

If you struggle with **test anxiety**, we strongly encourage you to check out our recommendations for how you can overcome it. Test anxiety is a formidable foe, but it can be beaten, and we want to make sure you have the tools you need to defeat it.

1

Secret Key #1 – Plan Big, Study Small

There's a lot riding on your performance. If you want to ace this test, you're going to need to keep your skills sharp and the material fresh in your mind. You need a plan that lets you review everything you need to know while still fitting in your schedule. We'll break this strategy down into three categories.

Information Organization

Start with the information you already have: the official test outline. From this, you can make a complete list of all the concepts you need to cover before the test. Organize these concepts into groups that can be studied together, and create a list of any related vocabulary you need to learn so you can brush up on any difficult terms. You'll want to keep this vocabulary list handy once you actually start studying since you may need to add to it along the way.

Time Management

Once you have your set of study concepts, decide how to spread them out over the time you have left before the test. Break your study plan into small, clear goals so you have a manageable task for each day and know exactly what you're doing. Then just focus on one small step at a time. When you manage your time this way, you don't need to spend hours at a time studying. Studying a small block of content for a short period each day helps you retain information better and avoid stressing over how much you have left to do. You can relax knowing that you have a plan to cover everything in time. In order for this strategy to be effective though, you have to start studying early and stick to your schedule. Avoid the exhaustion and futility that comes from last-minute cramming!

Study Environment

The environment you study in has a big impact on your learning. Studying in a coffee shop, while probably more enjoyable, is not likely to be as fruitful as studying in a quiet room. It's important to keep distractions to a minimum. You're only planning to study for a short block of time, so make the most of it. Don't pause to check your phone or get up to find a snack. It's also important to **avoid multitasking**. Research has consistently shown that multitasking will make your studying dramatically less effective. Your study area should also be comfortable and well-lit so you don't have the distraction of straining your eyes or sitting on an uncomfortable chair.

 The time of day you study is also important. You want to be rested and alert. Don't wait until just before bedtime. Study when you'll be most likely to comprehend and remember. Even better, if you know what time of day your test will be, set that time aside for study. That way your brain will be used to working on that subject at that specific time and you'll have a better chance of recalling information.

Finally, it can be helpful to team up with others who are studying for the same test. Your actual studying should be done in as isolated an environment as possible, but the work of organizing the information and setting up the study plan can be divided up. In between study sessions, you can discuss with your teammates the concepts that you're all studying and quiz each other on the details. Just be sure that your teammates are as serious about the test as you are. If you find that your study time is being replaced with social time, you might need to find a new team.

Secret Key #2 – Make Your Studying Count

You're devoting a lot of time and effort to preparing for this test, so you want to be absolutely certain it will pay off. This means doing more than just reading the content and hoping you can remember it on test day. It's important to make every minute of study count. There are two main areas you can focus on to make your studying count.

Retention

It doesn't matter how much time you study if you can't remember the material. You need to make sure you are retaining the concepts. To check your retention of the information you're learning, try recalling it at later times with minimal prompting. Try carrying around flashcards and glance at one or two from time to time or ask a friend who's also studying for the test to quiz you.

To enhance your retention, look for ways to put the information into practice so that you can apply it rather than simply recalling it. If you're using the information in practical ways, it will be much easier to remember. Similarly, it helps to solidify a concept in your mind if you're not only reading it to yourself but also explaining it to someone else. Ask a friend to let you teach them about a concept you're a little shaky on (or speak aloud to an imaginary audience if necessary). As you try to summarize, define, give examples, and answer your friend's questions, you'll understand the concepts better and they will stay with you longer. Finally, step back for a big picture view and ask yourself how each piece of information fits with the whole subject. When you link the different concepts together and see them working together as a whole, it's easier to remember the individual components.

Finally, practice showing your work on any multi-step problems, even if you're just studying. Writing out each step you take to solve a problem will help solidify the process in your mind, and you'll be more likely to remember it during the test.

Modality

Modality simply refers to the means or method by which you study. Choosing a study modality that fits your own individual learning style is crucial. No two people learn best in exactly the same way, so it's important to know your strengths and use them to your advantage.

For example, if you learn best by visualization, focus on visualizing a concept in your mind and draw an image or a diagram. Try color-coding your notes, illustrating them, or creating symbols that will trigger your mind to recall a learned concept. If you learn best by hearing or discussing information, find a study partner who learns the same way or read aloud to yourself. Think about how to put the information in your own words. Imagine that you are giving a lecture on the topic and record yourself so you can listen to it later.

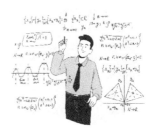

For any learning style, flashcards can be helpful. Organize the information so you can take advantage of spare moments to review. Underline key words or phrases. Use different colors for different categories. Mnemonic devices (such as creating a short list in which every item starts with the same letter) can also help with retention. Find what works best for you and use it to store the information in your mind most effectively and easily.

3

Secret Key #3 – Practice the Right Way

Your success on test day depends not only on how many hours you put into preparing, but also on whether you prepared the right way. It's good to check along the way to see if your studying is paying off. One of the most effective ways to do this is by taking practice tests to evaluate your progress. Practice tests are useful because they show exactly where you need to improve. Every time you take a practice test, pay special attention to these three groups of questions:

- The questions you got wrong
- The questions you had to guess on, even if you guessed right
- The questions you found difficult or slow to work through

This will show you exactly what your weak areas are, and where you need to devote more study time. Ask yourself why each of these questions gave you trouble. Was it because you didn't understand the material? Was it because you didn't remember the vocabulary? Do you need more repetitions on this type of question to build speed and confidence? Dig into those questions and figure out how you can strengthen your weak areas as you go back to review the material.

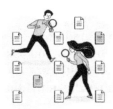 Additionally, many practice tests have a section explaining the answer choices. It can be tempting to read the explanation and think that you now have a good understanding of the concept. However, an explanation likely only covers part of the question's broader context. Even if the explanation makes perfect sense, **go back and investigate** every concept related to the question until you're positive you have a thorough understanding.

As you go along, keep in mind that the practice test is just that: practice. Memorizing these questions and answers will not be very helpful on the actual test because it is unlikely to have any of the same exact questions. If you only know the right answers to the sample questions, you won't be prepared for the real thing. **Study the concepts** until you understand them fully, and then you'll be able to answer any question that shows up on the test.

It's important to wait on the practice tests until you're ready. If you take a test on your first day of study, you may be overwhelmed by the amount of material covered and how much you need to learn. Work up to it gradually.

On test day, you'll need to be prepared for answering questions, managing your time, and using the test-taking strategies you've learned. It's a lot to balance, like a mental marathon that will have a big impact on your future. Like training for a marathon, you'll need to start slowly and work your way up. When test day arrives, you'll be ready.

Start with the strategies you've read in the first two Secret Keys—plan your course and study in the way that works best for you. If you have time, consider using multiple study resources to get different approaches to the same concepts. It can be helpful to see difficult concepts from more than one angle. Then find a good source for practice tests. Many times, the test website will suggest potential study resources or provide sample tests.

4

Practice Test Strategy

If you're able to find at least three practice tests, we recommend this strategy:

UNTIMED AND OPEN-BOOK PRACTICE

Take the first test with no time constraints and with your notes and study guide handy. Take your time and focus on applying the strategies you've learned.

TIMED AND OPEN-BOOK PRACTICE

Take the second practice test open-book as well, but set a timer and practice pacing yourself to finish in time.

TIMED AND CLOSED-BOOK PRACTICE

Take any other practice tests as if it were test day. Set a timer and put away your study materials. Sit at a table or desk in a quiet room, imagine yourself at the testing center, and answer questions as quickly and accurately as possible.

Keep repeating timed and closed-book tests on a regular basis until you run out of practice tests or it's time for the actual test. Your mind will be ready for the schedule and stress of test day, and you'll be able to focus on recalling the material you've learned.

Secret Key #4 – Pace Yourself

Once you're fully prepared for the material on the test, your biggest challenge on test day will be managing your time. Just knowing that the clock is ticking can make you panic even if you have plenty of time left. Work on pacing yourself so you can build confidence against the time constraints of the exam. Pacing is a difficult skill to master, especially in a high-pressure environment, so **practice is vital**.

Set time expectations for your pace based on how much time is available. For example, if a section has 60 questions and the time limit is 30 minutes, you know you have to average 30 seconds or less per question in order to answer them all. Although 30 seconds is the hard limit, set 25 seconds per question as your goal, so you reserve extra time to spend on harder questions. When you budget extra time for the harder questions, you no longer have any reason to stress when those questions take longer to answer.

Don't let this time expectation distract you from working through the test at a calm, steady pace, but keep it in mind so you don't spend too much time on any one question. Recognize that taking extra time on one question you don't understand may keep you from answering two that you do understand later in the test. If your time limit for a question is up and you're still not sure of the answer, mark it and move on, and come back to it later if the time and the test format allow. If the testing format doesn't allow you to return to earlier questions, just make an educated guess; then put it out of your mind and move on.

On the easier questions, be careful not to rush. It may seem wise to hurry through them so you have more time for the challenging ones, but it's not worth missing one if you know the concept and just didn't take the time to read the question fully. Work efficiently but make sure you understand the question and have looked at all of the answer choices, since more than one may seem right at first.

Even if you're paying attention to the time, you may find yourself a little behind at some point. You should speed up to get back on track, but do so wisely. Don't panic; just take a few seconds less on each question until you're caught up. Don't guess without thinking, but do look through the answer choices and eliminate any you know are wrong. If you can get down to two choices, it is often worthwhile to guess from those. Once you've chosen an answer, move on and don't dwell on any that you skipped or had to hurry through. If a question was taking too long, chances are it was one of the harder ones, so you weren't as likely to get it right anyway.

On the other hand, if you find yourself getting ahead of schedule, it may be beneficial to slow down a little. The more quickly you work, the more likely you are to make a careless mistake that will affect your score. You've budgeted time for each question, so don't be afraid to spend that time. Practice an efficient but careful pace to get the most out of the time you have.

6

Secret Key #5 – Have a Plan for Guessing

When you're taking the test, you may find yourself stuck on a question. Some of the answer choices seem better than others, but you don't see the one answer choice that is obviously correct. What do you do?

The scenario described above is very common, yet most test takers have not effectively prepared for it. Developing and practicing a plan for guessing may be one of the single most effective uses of your time as you get ready for the exam.

In developing your plan for guessing, there are three questions to address:

- When should you start the guessing process?
- How should you narrow down the choices?
- Which answer should you choose?

When to Start the Guessing Process

Unless your plan for guessing is to select C every time (which, despite its merits, is not what we recommend), you need to leave yourself enough time to apply your answer elimination strategies. Since you have a limited amount of time for each question, that means that if you're going to give yourself the best shot at guessing correctly, you have to decide quickly whether or not you will guess.

Of course, the best-case scenario is that you don't have to guess at all, so first, see if you can answer the question based on your knowledge of the subject and basic reasoning skills. Focus on the key words in the question and try to jog your memory of related topics. Give yourself a chance to bring the knowledge to mind, but once you realize that you don't have (or you can't access) the knowledge you need to answer the question, it's time to start the guessing process.

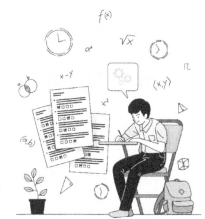

It's almost always better to start the guessing process too early than too late. It only takes a few seconds to remember something and answer the question from knowledge. Carefully eliminating wrong answer choices takes longer. Plus, going through the process of eliminating answer choices can actually help jog your memory.

Summary: Start the guessing process as soon as you decide that you can't answer the question based on your knowledge.

How to Narrow Down the Choices

The next chapter in this book (**Test-Taking Strategies**) includes a wide range of strategies for how to approach questions and how to look for answer choices to eliminate. You will definitely want to read those carefully, practice them, and figure out which ones work best for you. Here though, we're going to address a mindset rather than a particular strategy.

Your odds of guessing an answer correctly depend on how many options you are choosing from.

Number of options left	5	4	3	2	1
Odds of guessing correctly	20%	25%	33%	50%	100%

You can see from this chart just how valuable it is to be able to eliminate incorrect answers and make an educated guess, but there are two things that many test takers do that cause them to miss out on the benefits of guessing:

- Accidentally eliminating the correct answer
- Selecting an answer based on an impression

We'll look at the first one here, and the second one in the next section.

To avoid accidentally eliminating the correct answer, we recommend a thought exercise called **the $5 challenge**. In this challenge, you only eliminate an answer choice from contention if you are willing to bet $5 on it being wrong. Why $5? Five dollars is a small but not insignificant amount of money. It's an amount you could afford to lose but wouldn't want to throw away. And while losing $5 once might not hurt too much, doing it twenty times will set you back $100. In the same way, each small decision you make—eliminating a choice here, guessing on a question there—won't by itself impact your score very much, but when you put them all together, they can make a big difference. By holding each answer choice elimination decision to a higher standard, you can reduce the risk of accidentally eliminating the correct answer.

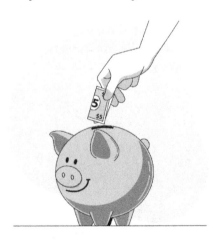

The $5 challenge can also be applied in a positive sense: If you are willing to bet $5 that an answer choice *is* correct, go ahead and mark it as correct.

Summary: Only eliminate an answer choice if you are willing to bet $5 that it is wrong.

Which Answer to Choose

You're taking the test. You've run into a hard question and decided you'll have to guess. You've eliminated all the answer choices you're willing to bet $5 on. Now you have to pick an answer. Why do we even need to talk about this? Why can't you just pick whichever one you feel like when the time comes?

The answer to these questions is that if you don't come into the test with a plan, you'll rely on your impression to select an answer choice, and if you do that, you risk falling into a trap. The test writers know that everyone who takes their test will be guessing on some of the questions, so they intentionally write wrong answer choices to seem plausible. You still have to pick an answer though, and if the wrong answer choices are designed to look right, how can you ever be sure that you're not falling for their trap? The best solution we've found to this dilemma is to take the decision out of your hands entirely. Here is the process we recommend:

Once you've eliminated any choices that you are confident (willing to bet $5) are wrong, select the first remaining choice as your answer.

Whether you choose to select the first remaining choice, the second, or the last, the important thing is that you use some preselected standard. Using this approach guarantees that you will not be enticed into selecting an answer choice that looks right, because you are not basing your decision on how the answer choices look.

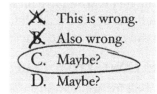

This is not meant to make you question your knowledge. Instead, it is to help you recognize the difference between your knowledge and your impressions. There's a huge difference between thinking an answer is right because of what you know, and thinking an answer is right because it looks or sounds like it should be right.

Summary: To ensure that your selection is appropriately random, make a predetermined selection from among all answer choices you have not eliminated.

Test-Taking Strategies

This section contains a list of test-taking strategies that you may find helpful as you work through the test. By taking what you know and applying logical thought, you can maximize your chances of answering any question correctly!

It is very important to realize that every question is different and every person is different: no single strategy will work on every question, and no single strategy will work for every person. That's why we've included all of them here, so you can try them out and determine which ones work best for different types of questions and which ones work best for you.

Question Strategies

⊘ READ CAREFULLY

Read the question and the answer choices carefully. Don't miss the question because you misread the terms. You have plenty of time to read each question thoroughly and make sure you understand what is being asked. Yet a happy medium must be attained, so don't waste too much time. You must read carefully and efficiently.

⊘ CONTEXTUAL CLUES

Look for contextual clues. If the question includes a word you are not familiar with, look at the immediate context for some indication of what the word might mean. Contextual clues can often give you all the information you need to decipher the meaning of an unfamiliar word. Even if you can't determine the meaning, you may be able to narrow down the possibilities enough to make a solid guess at the answer to the question.

⊘ PREFIXES

If you're having trouble with a word in the question or answer choices, try dissecting it. Take advantage of every clue that the word might include. Prefixes can be a huge help. Usually, they allow you to determine a basic meaning. *Pre-* means before, *post-* means after, *pro-* is positive, *de-* is negative. From prefixes, you can get an idea of the general meaning of the word and try to put it into context.

⊘ HEDGE WORDS

Watch out for critical hedge words, such as *likely, may, can, sometimes, often, almost, mostly, usually, generally, rarely,* and *sometimes.* Question writers insert these hedge phrases to cover every possibility. Often an answer choice will be wrong simply because it leaves no room for exception. Be on guard for answer choices that have definitive words such as *exactly* and *always.*

⊘ SWITCHBACK WORDS

Stay alert for *switchbacks.* These are the words and phrases frequently used to alert you to shifts in thought. The most common switchback words are *but, although,* and *however.* Others include *nevertheless, on the other hand, even though, while, in spite of, despite,* and *regardless of.* Switchback words are important to catch because they can change the direction of the question or an answer choice.

⊘ FACE VALUE

When in doubt, use common sense. Accept the situation in the problem at face value. Don't read too much into it. These problems will not require you to make wild assumptions. If you have to go beyond creativity and warp time or space in order to have an answer choice fit the question, then you should move on and consider the other answer choices. These are normal problems rooted in reality. The applicable relationship or explanation may not be readily apparent, but it is there for you to figure out. Use your common sense to interpret anything that isn't clear.

Answer Choice Strategies

⊘ ANSWER SELECTION

The most thorough way to pick an answer choice is to identify and eliminate wrong answers until only one is left, then confirm it is the correct answer. Sometimes an answer choice may immediately seem right, but be careful. The test writers will usually put more than one reasonable answer choice on each question, so take a second to read all of them and make sure that the other choices are not equally obvious. As long as you have time left, it is better to read every answer choice than to pick the first one that looks right without checking the others.

⊘ ANSWER CHOICE FAMILIES

An answer choice family consists of two (in rare cases, three) answer choices that are very similar in construction and cannot all be true at the same time. If you see two answer choices that are direct opposites or parallels, one of them is usually the correct answer. For instance, if one answer choice says that quantity x increases and another either says that quantity x decreases (opposite) or says that quantity y increases (parallel), then those answer choices would fall into the same family. An answer choice that doesn't match the construction of the answer choice family is more likely to be incorrect. Most questions will not have answer choice families, but when they do appear, you should be prepared to recognize them.

⊘ ELIMINATE ANSWERS

Eliminate answer choices as soon as you realize they are wrong, but make sure you consider all possibilities. If you are eliminating answer choices and realize that the last one you are left with is also wrong, don't panic. Start over and consider each choice again. There may be something you missed the first time that you will realize on the second pass.

⊘ AVOID FACT TRAPS

Don't be distracted by an answer choice that is factually true but doesn't answer the question. You are looking for the choice that answers the question. Stay focused on what the question is asking for so you don't accidentally pick an answer that is true but incorrect. Always go back to the question and make sure the answer choice you've selected actually answers the question and is not merely a true statement.

⊘ EXTREME STATEMENTS

In general, you should avoid answers that put forth extreme actions as standard practice or proclaim controversial ideas as established fact. An answer choice that states the "process should be used in certain situations, if…" is much more likely to be correct than one that states the "process should be discontinued completely." The first is a calm rational statement and doesn't even make a definitive, uncompromising stance, using a hedge word *if* to provide wiggle room, whereas the second choice is far more extreme.

⊘ Benchmark

As you read through the answer choices and you come across one that seems to answer the question well, mentally select that answer choice. This is not your final answer, but it's the one that will help you evaluate the other answer choices. The one that you selected is your benchmark or standard for judging each of the other answer choices. Every other answer choice must be compared to your benchmark. That choice is correct until proven otherwise by another answer choice beating it. If you find a better answer, then that one becomes your new benchmark. Once you've decided that no other choice answers the question as well as your benchmark, you have your final answer.

⊘ Predict the Answer

Before you even start looking at the answer choices, it is often best to try to predict the answer. When you come up with the answer on your own, it is easier to avoid distractions and traps because you will know exactly what to look for. The right answer choice is unlikely to be word-for-word what you came up with, but it should be a close match. Even if you are confident that you have the right answer, you should still take the time to read each option before moving on.

General Strategies

⊘ Tough Questions

If you are stumped on a problem or it appears too hard or too difficult, don't waste time. Move on! Remember though, if you can quickly check for obviously incorrect answer choices, your chances of guessing correctly are greatly improved. Before you completely give up, at least try to knock out a couple of possible answers. Eliminate what you can and then guess at the remaining answer choices before moving on.

⊘ Check Your Work

Since you will probably not know every term listed and the answer to every question, it is important that you get credit for the ones that you do know. Don't miss any questions through careless mistakes. If at all possible, try to take a second to look back over your answer selection and make sure you've selected the correct answer choice and haven't made a costly careless mistake (such as marking an answer choice that you didn't mean to mark). This quick double check should more than pay for itself in caught mistakes for the time it costs.

⊘ Pace Yourself

It's easy to be overwhelmed when you're looking at a page full of questions; your mind is confused and full of random thoughts, and the clock is ticking down faster than you would like. Calm down and maintain the pace that you have set for yourself. Especially as you get down to the last few minutes of the test, don't let the small numbers on the clock make you panic. As long as you are on track by monitoring your pace, you are guaranteed to have time for each question.

⊘ Don't Rush

It is very easy to make errors when you are in a hurry. Maintaining a fast pace in answering questions is pointless if it makes you miss questions that you would have gotten right otherwise. Test writers like to include distracting information and wrong answers that seem right. Taking a little extra time to avoid careless mistakes can make all the difference in your test score. Find a pace that allows you to be confident in the answers that you select.

⊘ Keep Moving

Panicking will not help you pass the test, so do your best to stay calm and keep moving. Taking deep breaths and going through the answer elimination steps you practiced can help to break through a stress barrier and keep your pace.

Final Notes

The combination of a solid foundation of content knowledge and the confidence that comes from practicing your plan for applying that knowledge is the key to maximizing your performance on test day. As your foundation of content knowledge is built up and strengthened, you'll find that the strategies included in this chapter become more and more effective in helping you quickly sift through the distractions and traps of the test to isolate the correct answer.

Now that you're preparing to move forward into the test content chapters of this book, be sure to keep your goal in mind. As you read, think about how you will be able to apply this information on the test. If you've already seen sample questions for the test and you have an idea of the question format and style, try to come up with questions of your own that you can answer based on what you're reading. This will give you valuable practice applying your knowledge in the same ways you can expect to on test day.

Good luck and good studying!

Safety and Compliance

Legal and Professional Considerations

ROLE OF LABORATORY PROFESSIONALS IN CUSTOMER SERVICE/SUPPORT

All laboratory professionals serve a role in customer service and support to some degree because they represent the organization with every patient contact, and the patient's attitude toward the organization may be based on this contact. The three components in any delivery of service are:

- The customer (patient, family member, or visitor)
- The organization (laboratory, hospitals)
- The individual service provider (lab professional)

For this reason, it is important that the individual remain professional, showing respect and consideration for the patient and others, maintaining a professional appearance, and carrying out duties competently. Communication is the essential element in customer service, including both conveying information in language appropriate to the listener and being an active listener. The laboratory professional should try to anticipate patient concerns, provide reassurance, and answer any questions in a positive, straightforward manner. Body language and words should both convey sincerity, and the laboratory professional should always handle complaints in a positive manner.

INTERPERSONAL COMMUNICATION WITH NON-LABORATORY PERSONNEL

Interpersonal communication skills are essential for the laboratory professional, who must interact with a variety of non-laboratory personnel in the work environment. Elements of effective communication include:

- Showing respect and consideration to others in all communications
- Recognizing each individual's scope of practice and responsibilities toward the patient
- Being an active listener, paying attention, and asking clarifying questions as necessary
- Sharing important information with the appropriate personnel
- Asking questions when in need of more information about a patient
- Ensuring that information is shared accurately
- Providing timely communication
- Discussing special needs of patients in relation to collection of a sample and processing
- Communicating any problems encountered with collection or processing with the appropriate personnel
- Discussing timing issues related to sample collection, such as STAT orders or collection that must be done at a specific time
- Scheduling collection to avoid interrupting other patient care activities when possible

MEDICARE HEALTH PLANS

Medicare Health Plans include managed care plans such as Medicare Advantage, cost plans, and healthcare prepayment plans. Services provided by contract providers (those who participate in these plans) are reimbursed by Medicare. However, non-contract providers—those outside of these plans who provide services to enrollees (patients), such as a laboratory—may not be reimbursed. If Medicare denies payment to a non-contract provider, that provider must receive notice regarding the reason for the denial and the steps to appeal the decision. The filing for reconsideration must be done within 60 days from the date of notification and must include a signed **waiver of liability**

15

form. The form contains the enrollee's Medicare number and name, the name of the non-contract provider, the dates of service, and the name of the health plan. The waiver of liability statement waives any right to collect payment for the services provided regardless of the outcome of the appeal process, although the provider maintains the right to further appeal.

LIABILITY

Liability is legal responsibility for something an individual has done or failed to do. Elements of liability include:

- **Neglect**: Failure to provide basic needs or usual standards of care or exhibiting an uncaring attitude toward a patient
- **Abandonment**: A unilateral severing of the professional relationship between the healthcare provider and the patient with no notice that would allow the patient to make other arrangements
- **Assault**: A threat to touch another person against the patient's will, such as threatening to withdraw blood from an uncooperative patient
- **Battery**: Following through with a threat and touching another person without consent, such as forcing the patient to undergo venipuncture
- **Tort**: A negligent act that causes injury or suffering to another person and is the basis for a civil action, such as a lawsuit
- **Malpractice**: Failure to meet standards of care or wrongfully carrying out duties in such a way as to bring harm to a patient

PATIENT CONSENT

Patients should provide **informed consent** prior to any procedures, including laboratory tests. That is, the patient should understand the purpose, the risks, and the benefits, as well as the method that will be used in the procedure. Hospitalized patients sign a general consent form that covers most routine laboratory tests, although some tests, such as HIV tests, may require a separate consent form. While consent may be verbal or in writing, written consent provides the most protection for the healthcare provider. Competent adult patients have the **right to refuse any treatment**, even if it is lifesaving. If a patient refuses a test (for example, a blood draw), the phlebotomist must immediately stop, inform the ordering healthcare provider, and document the refusal.

TYPES OF PATIENT CONSENT

The types of patient consent include the following:

- **Informed consent**: A competent person is able to provide voluntary permission for a medical procedure after receiving adequate information about the risk, methods used, and consequences of the procedure.
- **Expressed consent**: This is permission given by the patient, verbally or in writing, for a procedure.
- **Implied consent**: The patient's actions imply permission for the procedure without verbal or written consent, for example, going to the emergency room to receive care, or holding out an arm when told of the need to draw blood.
- **HIV consent**: Special permission must be granted to administer a test for detecting the human immunodeficiency virus.
- **Parental consent for minors**: A parent or a legal guardian must give permission for procedures administered to underage patients. Depending on the state law, the patient may be considered underage if they are younger than 21 or younger than 18.

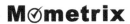

Point-of-Care Testing, Laboratory Procedures, and Phlebotomy

OCCUPATIONAL SAFETY AND HEALTH ADMINISTRATION (OSHA)

The Occupational Safety and Health Administration (OSHA) is an organization designed to ensure the safety and health of workers by setting and enforcing standards; providing training, outreach, and education; establishing partnerships; and encouraging continual improvement in workplace safety and health.

SDS (formerly MSDS) stands for **Safety Data Sheets**. These sheets are the result of the "Right to Know" Law, also known as OSHA's Hazard Communication Standard (HCS). This law requires chemical manufacturers to supply SDS sheets on any products that have a hazardous warning label. These sheets contain information on precautionary as well as emergency information about the product.

> **Review Video: Intro to OSHA**
> Visit mometrix.com/academy and enter code: 913559

OSHA REGULATIONS REGARDING LABORATORY SERVICES

OSHA requires that facilities provide safe medical equipment and devices. OSHA also regulates workplace safety, including disposal methods for sharps, such as needles, and blood disposition. OSHA requires that standard precautions be used at all times and that staff be trained to use precautions. OSHA requires procedures for post-exposure evaluation and treatment and availability of hepatitis B vaccine for healthcare workers. OSHA defines occupational exposure to infections, establishes standards to prevent the spread of bloodborne pathogens, and regulates the fitting and use of respirators. OSHA requires the use of needleless blood transfer devices as a means of decreasing the risk of needlestick injuries and infection as part of OSHA's Bloodborne Pathogen Standard. Sharps used for blood draw should have sharps injury protection devices whenever possible. Needles without this protection should never be recapped, as this increases risk of needlestick. States may have their own OSHA-approved programs but must meet the minimum standards developed by OSHA.

LABORATORY STANDARDS AND INTEGRITY ASSESSMENT

Laboratory standards are established by a number of agencies, including OSHA, which establishes safety standards; the EPA, which established good laboratory practices; CLSI, which provides global laboratory standards; and ISO-9000, which establishes standards for quality management. Laboratory standards are norms or requirements established for the profession. **Integrity assessment** is carried out to determine if a laboratory is meeting standards or has engaged in fraud or misconduct (as opposed to accidents or errors), such as through:

- Failure to properly carry out procedures
- Falsification of records or measurements, incomplete documentation, manipulation of data
- Violation of standards or rules of conduct, violations of codes of ethics
- Misrepresentation of quality assurance results
- Failure to adequately calibrate equipment
- Failure to retain samples for the required time
- Improper storage of reagents, samples, and supplies
- Failure to follow standard operating procedures
- Alterations of log book
- Employment of personnel without appropriate license or certification

Integrity assessment may include reviewing data, comparing manual logs with computer logs, conducting an audit trail, carrying out unannounced audits, and encouraging and supporting whistleblowers.

GOVERNMENTAL AND NONGOVERNMENTAL REGULATORY ENTITIES

The **Clinical and Laboratory Standards Institute (CLSI)** provides standards for a wide range of performance and testing and covers all types of laboratory functions and microbiology. These standards are used as a basis for quality control procedures. Standards include: labeling, security/information technology, toxicology/drug testing, statistical quality control, and performance standards for various types of antimicrobial susceptibility testing.

In the United States, all laboratory testing, except for research, is regulated by the CMS (Centers for Medicare and Medicaid) through the **Clinical Laboratory Improvement Amendments (CLIA)**. CLIA is implemented through the Division of Laboratory Services and serves approximately 244,000 laboratories. Laboratories receiving reimbursement from CMS must meet CLIA standards, which ensure that laboratory testing will be accurate and procedures followed properly.

The **Centers for Disease Control and Prevention (CDC)** is a federal agency that supports health promotion, prevention, and health preparedness. The CDC partners with CMS and the FDA in supporting CLIA programs.

The **National Accrediting Agency for Clinical Laboratory Sciences** is responsible for approving and accrediting clinical laboratory science and similar healthcare professional education programs.

The **College of American Pathologists** is the primary organization for board-certified pathologists serving to represent the interests of the public, as well as pathologists and their patients, by fostering excellence in the pathology and laboratory medicine practice.

The **Joint Commission** is a large organization that aims to improve the quality of care provided to patients through implementing healthcare accreditation standards and other supportive services aimed at improving the performance of healthcare organizations.

ADA SAFETY REGULATIONS FOR LABORATORIES

According to the American with Disabilities Act's laboratory safety regulations, the following guidelines must be adhered to:

- Workstations must be adjustable (28–34 inches in height and 27 inches of knee clearance) so they are accessible to individuals who use wheelchairs or other assistive devices.
- Floors must be free of clutter.
- Fume heads, sinks, and emergency showers must be accessible with the controls within reach of persons in wheelchairs.
- Eyewash stations and showers must be accessible within 10 seconds of injury, any door separating the workspace from the eyewash stations and showers must open in the direction of traffic, and no obstructions should be located within 16 inches of the center of the shower spray.
- Doorways must be at least 32 inches wide to accommodate wheelchairs, and room must be available for wheelchairs to turn 360° with aisle width up to 60 inches.
- Alarms must be both audio and visual, and evacuation protocols must accommodate individuals with various types of disabilities.
- Signage must accommodate persons with vision impairment (e.g., by using braille or tactile characters).

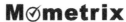

SPECIMEN COLLECTION STANDARDS

The Clinical and Laboratory Standards Institute provides standards and procedures for specimen collection, including the following:

- **Patient preparation**: Fasting requirements and required instructions.
- **Procedures**: Details about collecting different types of specimens.
- **Labels**: Labeling should be done in the presence of the patient and must contain the patient's name, the patient-specific identifier, the patient's date of birth, the date and time of collection, additional pertinent information (e.g., whether the patient is fasting or non-fasting), and the initials of the phlebotomist.
- **Puncture devices**: The sterility and appropriateness of the device must be ensured. Some regulations exist for specific types of puncture devices, procedures, and depths, including those for capillary punctures.
- **Evacuated tubes**: Color-coded tubes must be sterile and have expiration dates and lot numbers so they can be easily tracked.

The Joint Commission has similar guidelines as part of their laboratory services accreditation process. It has established strict protocols for patient identification (e.g., using two patient identifiers) and requires that appropriate personal protective equipment be used. Orders must be clearly documented for each specimen obtained, and specimens must be obtained in accordance with established protocols.

SPECIMEN SHIPPING REGULATIONS

The Department of Transportation and the International Air Transport Association have established regulations for the shipping of specimens that may be infectious or hazardous. Regulations classify biological substances into two categories, as follows:

- **Category A**: Substances capable of causing permanent disability or life-threatening disease in animals and humans. They must be triple packaged in containers that can withstand shocks, changes in pressure, and other conditions. Labels must contain a United Nations (UN) number, an infectious substance label, and a biohazard symbol. Handling documents may also be required, and a "shipper's declaration for dangerous goods" form must be completed. The carrier must be approved to carry category A specimens.
- **Category B**: Non-category A substances that may cause non-life-threatening infection. They must be triple packaged in watertight containers (e.g., plastic, metal, or glass) with positive closure, and they must be labeled with the shipping name (e.g., "Biological substance, category B"). The label must also include the UN number and must display the biohazard symbol. If ice or dry ice is used, it must be outside the secondary container, and dry ice must be labeled as class 9. Specimens may not exceed 500 mL or 500 g. Documentation, such as a waybill, must accompany the specimen and must include the name and access information for a person responsible for the shipment. The carrier must be approved to carry category B specimens.

STANDARDS FOR CODING/BILLING

INTERNATIONAL CLASSIFICATION OF DISEASES (ICD)

The World Health Organization developed the **International Classification of Diseases** (ICD). In January 2022, ICD-11 took effect and replaced ICD-10 CM. In ICD-11, alphanumeric codes are used for diagnoses, and it provide data regarding mortality and morbidity. ICD-11 links with other terminology (such as that from the Systematized Nomenclature of Medicine). The ICD-10 Procedure

Coding System (PCS), on the other hand, was developed by the Centers for Medicare and Medicaid Services (CMS) to code for inpatient hospital procedures, and ICD-10 PCS remains current.

ICD-10 PCS codes comprise seven characters that provide information about seven different items, in order as follows: section, body system, operation, body part, approach, device, and qualifier. For example, 0HBT0ZX is the code for a diagnostic open excision of the right breast:

Section	0	Medical and Surgical
Body system	H	Skin and Breast
Operation	B	Excision
Body part	T	Breast, Right
Approach	0	Open
Device	Z	No device
Qualifier	X	Diagnostic

However, for laboratory tests, hospitals typically use Current Procedural Terminology codes, which are developed and published by the American Medical Association, with codes ranging from 80047 to 89398. For example, the code for a complete blood count with automated differential is 85025.

TEST COMPLEXITY

Laboratory tests are categorized by the Food and Drug Administration according to their level of test complexity, which is reflected in their billing codes and reimbursement. Tests with higher complexity face more stringent Clinical Laboratory Improvement Amendments requirements. To determine complexity, a seven-item scorecard is used, with each item scored as 1 for low complexity, 2 for intermediate complexity, or 3 for high complexity. The seven items are (1) knowledge; (2) training and experience; (3) reagents and materials preparation; (4) characteristics of operational steps; (5) calibration, quality control, and proficiency testing materials; (6) test system troubleshooting and equipment maintenance; and (7) interpretation and judgment.

- **Waived tests**: These tests can be purchased over the counter, are used in the home environment, and pose no risk to the user, such as testing urine with a dipstick.
- **Moderate-complexity tests**: These tests are relatively easy to perform and pose minimal risk, such as a complete blood count.
- **High-complexity tests**: These tests require higher standards, more training, and more frequent quality control assessment (e.g., polymerase chain reaction testing).

CMS ADVANCE BENEFICIARY NOTICE OF NON-COVERAGE (ABN)

An Advance Beneficiary Notice of Non-coverage (ABN) (Form CMS-R-131) is given to original Medicare and Medicare fee-for-service patients (not Medicare managed care or private fee-for-service patients) by healthcare providers to notify them that an item or service is not covered by Medicare (usually meaning that supplementary insurance will also not cover the item or service). An ABN may also be issued if a patient wants a service or item that is not deemed medically necessary at that time but is a service or item that is generally covered by Medicare. ABNs are not required to inform patients of services that are never covered by Medicare, such as acupuncture. For those on Medicare Advantage plans, CMS does not require that the patient be provided an ABN for noncovered items or services, but the healthcare provider may do so as a courtesy to alert patients. When ABNs are provided on a voluntary basis to notify patients of noncovered items/services, patients should not sign the form, nor should they indicate a choice of the options given.

SOP FOR LABORATORIES

Each laboratory should draw up a **standard operating procedure (SOP) document** that outlines all the processes and procedures associated with the reception of a sample and processing, including:

- **Specimen collection processes**: PPE, patient identification, collection tubes, collecting procedures, need for special handling, labeling, transporting specimens, criteria for rejecting inadequate samples, protocols for adverse reactions
- **Chain of custody**: Labeling, storing, packing, and transporting
- **Sample reception**: Specimen identification, logging, specimen condition, specimen accountability, retention times
- **Rejection criteria**: Incorrect collection tube, leaking tube, incorrect labeling, incorrect sample for test, volume inadequate, order unverified, mismatch between order and labeling
- **Delivery** (from reception to processing): Process for delivery to correct department, specimen retention policies
- **Processing**: Procedures for testing, accountability standards, storage, and retention policies
- **Reporting**: Methods of reporting and timeframes

Laboratory Safety and Quality Control

QUALITY IMPROVEMENT

Quality improvement is a systematic method of analyzing performance and improving the quality of performance, usually across an entire organization, although more localized quality improvement methods may be employed. Methods of quality improvement include:

- **Continuous Quality Improvement** (CQI): Emphasizes the organization, and systems and processes within that organization, rather than individuals. It recognizes internal customers (staff) and external customers (patients) and uses data to improve processes.
- **Total Quality Management** (TQM): Espouses a commitment to meeting the needs of the customers at all levels within an organization, promoting not only continuous improvement but also a dedication to quality in all aspects of an organization. Outcomes should include increased customer satisfaction, productivity, and increased profits through efficiency and reduction in costs.
- **Six Sigma**: A data-driven performance model that aims to eliminate "defects" in processes that involve products or services. The first model for Six Sigma is DMAIC (define, measure, analyze, improve, control), which is used when existing processes or products need improvement; it is used in healthcare quality.

PHILOSOPHY OF CONTINUOUS QUALITY IMPROVEMENT

Continuous quality improvement is a multidisciplinary management philosophy that can be applied to all aspects of an organization, including those related to such varied areas as the cardiac unit, purchasing, laboratories, or human resources. The skills used for epidemiologic research (data collection, analysis, outcomes, action plans) are all applicable to analysis of multiple types of events because they are based on solid scientific methods. Multidisciplinary planning can bring valuable insights from various perspectives, and strategies used in one context can often be applied to another. All staff, from housekeeping to supervising, must be alert to not only problems but also opportunities for improvement. Increasingly, departments must be concerned with cost-effectiveness as the costs of medical care continue to rise, so the quality professional in the cardiovascular unit is not in an isolated position in an institution but is just one part of the whole, facing concerns similar to those in other disciplines. Disciplines are often interrelated in their functions.

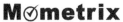

DEMING'S 14 POINTS FOR QUALITY IMPROVEMENT

W. Edwards Deming was an author and statistician who developed several models for cataloging and determining quality. His 14 points for quality improvement are used throughout many industries.

- Create and communicate to all employees a statement of the quality philosophy of the company.
- Adopt this philosophy.
- Build quality into a product throughout production.
- End the practice of awarding business on the basis of price tag alone, and build a long-term relationship based on established loyalty and trust.
- Work to constantly improve quality and productivity.
- Institute on-the-job quality training.
- Teach and institute leadership to improve all job functions.
- Drive out fear, create trust.
- Strive to reduce inter- and intradepartmental conflicts.
- Eliminate slogans and targets. Instead, focus on the system and morale.
- Eliminate numerical quotas for production and management. Substitute leadership methods for improvement.
- Remove barriers that rob people of pride in their work.
- Educate with self-improvement programs.
- Include everyone in the company to accomplish the transformation.

RISK MANAGEMENT

Risk management attempts to prevent harm and legal liability by being proactive and by identifying a patient's **risk factors**. The patient should be educated about these factors and ways that they can modify their behavior to decrease their risk. Treatments and interventions must be considered in terms of risk to the patient, and the patient must always know these risks in order to make healthcare decisions. Much can be done to avoid mistakes that put patients at risk. Patients should note medications, allergies, and other aspects of their care so that they can help prevent mistakes. They should feel free to question care and to have their concerns heard and addressed. When mistakes are made, the actions taken to remedy the situation are very important. The physician or nurse should be made aware of the error immediately, and the patient notified according to hospital policy. Errors must be evaluated to determine how the process failed. Honesty and caring can help mitigate many errors.

Laboratory Infection Control

CHAIN OF INFECTION

In order for an infection to spread, it requires an agent, a host, and the proper environment (known as the epidemiologic triad). The **chain of infection** takes that model a step further, stating that in order for a pathogenic microorganism to leave its original reservoir (which could be an animal, a human, or the environment), it needs the following:

- A portal of exit from that reservoir
- A susceptible host to inhabit
- A mode of transmission between reservoir and host
- A portal of entry into the host

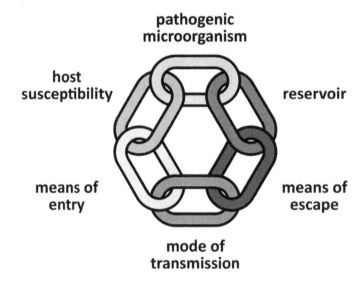

BASIC INFECTION CONTROL MEASURES

Standard infection control measures are designed to prevent transmission of microbial substances between patients and/or medical providers. These measures are indicated for everyone and include frequent handwashing, gloves whenever bodily fluids are involved, and face shields and gowns when splashes are anticipated.

For more advanced control with tuberculosis, SARS, vesicular rash disorders (such as VZV), and (more recently) COVID-19, **airborne precautions** should be instituted to prevent the spread of tiny droplets that can remain suspended in the air for days and travel throughout a hospital environment. Therefore, negative pressure rooms are essential, and providers and patients should wear high-efficiency N95 masks and be fitted in advance.

For disorders such as influenza or other infections spread by droplets (spread by cough or sneeze) **droplet precautions** such as wearing basic surgical masks must be taken.

For **contact precautions** in the setting of fecally transmitted infection or vesicular rash diseases, gowns/gloves should be used and contact limited. White coats are not a substitute for proper gowning.

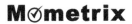

DIRECT AND INDIRECT CONTACT TRANSMISSION

According to the CDC, contact transmission is the most common form of disease transmission. Organisms commonly spread through contact include herpes simplex, *Clostridioides difficile,* and *Staphylococcus aureus.* Types of contact transmission:

- **Direct contact**: Transmission is directly from one person to another, usually because of touch. Examples include a person's blood or other body fluids entering broken skin, mucous membranes, or the cuts of another person (such as with HIV), as well as mites (such as scabies) from one person transferring to another's skin.
- **Indirect contact**: Transmission occurs from one person, through an intermediary object or person, and then to another person. Examples include when a caregiver's hands touch a patient or bedrails contaminated with a pathogen and then pass that pathogen to a third person (such as with *Clostridioides difficile*), and when patient care devices or other items are shared among different patients.

PROPER INFECTION CONTROL PRECAUTIONS

Each laboratory should carry out a biological risk assessment every year or when new risks arise to determine the biosafety level, agent hazards, and procedure hazards. Work practices should conform to the Bloodborne Pathogen Standard (OSHA) and standard precautions (CDC). **Infection control precautions** include:

- Using appropriate hand hygiene, with a hands-free sink for washing hands available near exit
- Using mechanical pipettes instead of mouth pipetting
- Prohibiting eating, drinking, smoking, storing food, applying makeup, and handling contact lenses in the laboratory
- Maintaining policies for the safe handling of sharps
- Using safety devices (retractable needles, lances) when possible
- Minimizing splashing or aerosolizing liquids
- Decontaminating potentially infectious materials prior to disposal
- Packing potentially infectious materials for disposal outside of the facility in appropriate packaging according to regulations
- Maintaining a pest management program
- Ensuring that all personnel are adequately trained
- Ensuring appropriate immunizations and screening for personnel
- Making PPE available and monitoring appropriate use
- Ensuring that an eye wash station is easily accessible and available

SPECIFIC INFECTION PREVENTION AND CONTROL

HEPATITIS B

The hepatitis B virus (HBV) and its exposure hazards are discussed below:

- Hepatitis B is a sexually transmitted infection, also transmitted with body fluids.
- Some individuals may be symptom free but still be carriers.
- Condoms are not proven to prevent the spread of this disease.
- Symptoms include jaundice, dark urine, malaise, joint pain, fever, and fatigue.
- Labs will show decreased albumin levels, positive hepatitis B antibodies and antigens, and increased levels of transaminase.
- For treatment, monitor for changes in the liver. Recombinant interferon alpha may be used in some cases. Transplant is necessary if liver failure occurs.
- Prevention involves a series of three hepatitis B vaccinations: an initial dose, a dose 1 month later, and a final dose 6 months after the initial dose.
- HBV is the most common laboratory-associated infection.

HEPATITIS D

The hepatitis D virus (HDV) is the most severe form of hepatitis. It occurs in the presence of hepatitis B. Its exposure hazards are discussed below:

- Hepatitis D, also referred to as delta hepatitis, involves severe infection of the liver. It requires hepatitis B to replicate and therefore occurs as a superinfection with hepatitis B. Without hepatitis B, hepatitis D cannot thrive.
- Signs and symptoms include jaundice, fatigue, abdominal pain, loss of appetite, nausea, vomiting, joint pain, and dark (tea-colored) urine.
- Transmission occurs when blood from an infected person enters the body of a person who is not immune. This can happen through sharing drugs injected by needles; through needlesticks or sharps exposures on the job; or from an infected mother to her baby during birth. Activation and replication of hepatitis D then occurs in the individual with hepatitis B.
- Treatment for acute HDV infection involves supportive care. Treatment for chronic HDV infection involves interferon alpha and liver transplant.
- Because hepatitis D requires hepatitis B to replicate, prevention of hepatitis D is through the prevention of HBV with hepatitis B vaccination. For individuals who already have HBV, prevention of hepatitis D is through education to reduce high-risk behaviors and avoid transmission.

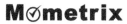

HIV

The following are ways that HIV can be **transmitted** from an infected person to an uninfected one:

- HIV can be transmitted through **direct blood contact**, including injection-drug needles, blood transfusions, accidents in healthcare settings, or use of certain blood products.
- **Sexual intercourse (vaginal and anal)**: In the genitals and the rectum, HIV may infect the mucous membranes directly or enter through cuts and sores caused during intercourse (many of which would be unnoticed).
- **Oral sex** (mouth-penis, mouth-vagina): The mouth is an inhospitable environment for HIV (HIV is more often found in semen, vaginal fluid, or blood), meaning the risk of HIV transmission through the throat, gums, and oral membranes is lower than through vaginal or anal membranes. There are, however, documented cases where HIV was transmitted orally.
- **Sharing injection needles**: An injection needle can pass blood directly from one person's bloodstream to another. It is a very efficient way to transmit a bloodborne virus.
- **Mother to child**: It is possible for an HIV-infected mother to pass the virus directly before or during birth, or through breast milk. The following bodily fluids are *not* infectious: saliva, tears, sweat, feces, and urine.

PROTOCOL FOR NEEDLESTICK INJURY

If the phlebotomist experiences a needlestick injury after carrying out a venipuncture, the phlebotomist's initial response should be to wash the wound with soap and water. As soon as possible, the incident must be reported to a supervisor, and steps should be taken according to established protocol. This may include testing and/or prophylaxis, depending on the patient's health history. In some cases, the patient may also be tested for communicable diseases, such as HIV, in order to determine the risk to the phlebotomist. PEP (post-exposure prophylaxis) is available for exposure to HIV and HBV. However, no PEP is available for HCV (hepatitis C virus), although the CDC does provide a plan for management. PEP should be initiated within 72 hours of exposure. All testing and treatments associated with the needlestick injury must be provided free of cost to the phlebotomist.

DONNING AND DOFFING PROTECTIVE CLOTHING

A healthcare worker puts on (dons) the protective gown first, being sure not to touch the outside of the gown. The mask is put on next. Gloves are applied last and are secured over the cuffs of the gown. When doffing (taking off) protective clothing, a healthcare worker removes the gloves first. They are removed by grasping one glove at the wrist and pulling it inside out, off the hand, and holding it in the gloved hand. The second glove is removed by placing the uncovered hand's fingers under the edge of the glove, being careful not to touch the outside of the glove, and rolling it down inside out over the glove grasped in the gloved hand. The first glove ends up inside of the second glove. Next, slide your arms out of the gown, and then fold the gown with the outside folded away from the body so that the contaminated side is folded inwardly. Dispose of properly. Finally, remove the mask by touching the strings only. Always wash hands after glove removal.

27

Laboratory Hazards

BIOLOGICAL/BIOHAZARDOUS AND HAZARDOUS WASTE

Biological wastes are those that contain or are contaminated with pathogens (human, plant, animal); rDNA; blood, cell, or tissue products; or cultures. Biological wastes that are, or may be, infectious or rDNA contaminated (biohazardous waste) must be inactivated before disposal in hazardous waste containers. Typically, inactivation is carried out with autoclaving or treating with hypochlorite solution (bleach). Contaminated sharps must be maintained in special sharps containers to avoid injury to handlers, and they must be inactivated before disposal. Non-infectious biological wastes, such as uncontaminated gloves, do not require deactivation and are disposed of in biological waste containers.

Biohazard Symbol

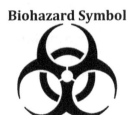

Hazardous wastes—those that are ignitable, corrosive, reactive, or toxic—are any that are harmful to humans or the environment. They may be solids, liquids, gases, or sludges. Hazardous wastes are generally transported by hazardous waste transporters in special hazardous waste containers to treatment, storage, and disposal facilities (TSDFs), where they are stored, inactivated, and/or recycled.

ROUTES BIOLOGICAL HAZARDS MAY TAKE TO ENTER THE BODY

Biological hazards may enter the body through the following avenues:

- Airborne (through the nasal passage into the lungs)
- Ingestion (by eating)
- Broken skin
- Percutaneous (through intact skin)
- Mucosal (through the lining of the mouth and nose)

CLEANING UP SMALL BLOOD SPILLS

The best way to clean a small blood spill is to absorb the blood with a paper towel or gauze pad. Then disinfect the area with a disinfectant. Soap and water are not considered disinfectants, nor is alcohol. Never scrape a dry spill; this may cause an aerosol of infectious organisms. If blood is dried, use the disinfectant to moisten the dried blood.

PROTOCOL FOR THE DISPOSAL OF REAGENTS

Laboratories use many different reagent solutions, which comprise a solid (solute) dissolved in a liquid (solvent). The three most common **types of reagents** are:

- **Stock**: Concentrate that is diluted to prepare a working solution
- **Working**: Diluted solution ready for use
- **Standard**: Reference solution used to identify the concentration of other solutions

Reagents may be classified as solid wastes (which can include liquids) or hazardous wastes. Some reagents, such as those containing sodium azide, must be disposed of as hazardous waste in hazardous waste drums and sent to hazardous waste facilities for incineration (most hazardous wastes cannot go into landfills). But some other reagents, such as ethanol diluted to less than 24%, may be discharged into the sewer. Some, such as DAB (3,3'-diaminobenzidine), may be detoxified before sewer disposal. Manufacturer's directions for disposal must be followed for each reagent.

BIOTERRORISM

Bioterrorism is the use of biological agents (viruses, bacteria, fungi) to attack and cause illness, death, or contamination in people, air supplies, water supplies, animals, or crops. There are similar steps to take regardless of the pathogen. An organized approach should include the following steps:

- Be on the alert for possible bioterrorism-related infections, based on clusters of patients or symptoms.
- Use personal protection equipment, including respirators when indicated.
- Complete a thorough assessment of the patient, including medical history, physical examination, immunization record, and travel history.
- The physician should give a probable diagnosis based on symptoms and lab findings, including cultures.
- Healthcare staff should provide treatment, including prophylaxis while waiting for laboratory findings.
- Use transmission precautions as well as isolation for suspected biologic agents.
- Notify local, state, and federal authorities per established protocol.
- Conduct surveillance and epidemiological studies to identify at-risk populations.
- Healthcare facilities should develop plans to accommodate large numbers of patients, such as:
  o Restricting elective admissions
  o Transferring patients to other facilities
  o Reusing existing facilities

FIRE SAFETY

Fire requires three components, known as the fire triangle, in order to occur. The fire triangle consists of fuel, oxygen, and heat. When a chemical source is included, it is known as the fire tetrahedron.

Fires are broken down into **five classes**:

- Class A fires involve ordinary combustible materials.
- Class B fires involve flammable liquids.
- Class C fires are electrical fires.
- Class D fires involve combustible metals.
- Class K fires involve oils or fats.

In the event of a fire, remember these two acronyms: RACE (steps for dealing with the situation) and PASS (proper use of a fire extinguisher).

Rescue	Rescue patients and co-workers from danger.	**P**ull the pin.
Alarm	Sound the alarm and alert those around you.	**A**im at the fire.
Confine	Confine a fire by closing the doors and windows.	**S**queeze the trigger.
Extinguish	Use the nearest fire extinguisher to put out the fire.	**S**weep the base of the fire.

Ethics

ETHICAL PRINCIPLES

Autonomy is the ethical principle that the individual has the right to make decisions about his or her own care. In the case of children or patients with dementia who cannot make autonomous decisions, parents or family members may serve as the legal decision-makers. The healthcare worker must keep the patient and/or family fully informed so that they can exercise their autonomy in informed decision-making.

Justice is the ethical principle that relates to the distribution of the limited resources of healthcare benefits to the members of society. These resources must be distributed fairly. For example, imagine there is only one bed left, but two sick patients. Justice comes into play in deciding which patient should stay and which should be transported or otherwise cared for. The decision should be made according to what is best or most just for the patients and not colored by personal bias.

Beneficence is an ethical principle that involves performing actions for the purpose of benefiting another person. In the care of a patient, any procedure or treatment should be done with the ultimate goal of benefiting the patient, and any actions that are not beneficial should be reconsidered. As conditions change, procedures need to be continually reevaluated to determine if they are still of benefit.

Nonmaleficence is an ethical principle that means healthcare workers should provide care in a manner that does not cause direct intentional harm to the patient:

- The actual act must be good or morally neutral.
- The intent must be only for a good effect.
- A bad effect cannot serve as the means to get to a good effect.
- A good effect's benefit must be greater than a bad effect's harm.

SCOPE OF PRACTICE AND ETHICAL STANDARDS RELATED TO PRACTICE OF PHLEBOTOMY

The **scope of practice** encompasses those duties and procedures that the person's training, licensure, and/or certification have prepared the person to undertake. The phlebotomist and other laboratory professionals must adhere to the **code of ethics** developed by the American Society for Clinical Laboratory Sciences (ASCLS):

- **Duty to patient**: This is the primary focus and depends on being honest, showing respect for the patient, and providing a high standard of care.
- **Duty to colleagues and profession**: The phlebotomist and laboratory professionals must establish an honest and cooperative working relationship with colleagues and work to improve personal practice and to advance the profession.
- **Duty to society**: The phlebotomist and laboratory professionals must comply with laws and regulations and serve as patient advocates.
- **Pledge**: The phlebotomist and laboratory professionals pledge to carry out the duties outlined in the code of ethics, beginning with placing the welfare of the patient before that of self.

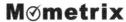

BIOETHICS

Bioethics is a branch of ethics that involves making sure that the medical treatment given is the most morally correct choice given the different options that might be available and the differences inherent in the varied levels of treatment. In the healthcare unit, if the patients, family members, and staff are in agreement when it comes to values and decision-making, then no ethical dilemma exists; however, when there is a difference in value beliefs between the patients/family members and the staff, there is a bioethical dilemma that must be resolved. Sometimes, discussion and explanation can resolve differences, but at times the institution's ethics committee must be brought in to resolve the conflict. The primary goal of bioethics is to determine the most morally correct action using the set of circumstances given.

ETHICAL ANALYSIS OF A SITUATION

Assessment of the situation reveals the **ethical, legal, and professional conflicts** that are present. Those who are involved are identified, including the patient, family, and healthcare personnel. The decision-maker is determined if it is not the patient. Information about the situation is collected to determine medical facts about the disease and condition of the patient, options for treatment, and diagnoses. Any pertinent legal information is included. The patient and family's cultural, religious, and moral values are determined. Possible courses of action are listed and compared in terms of outcomes for the patient using the utilitarian or deontological theory of ethics. Professional codes of ethics are also applied. A decision is made and evaluated as to whether it is the most morally correct action. Ethical arguments for and against the decision are given and responded to by the decision-maker.

PATIENT RIGHTS AND RESPONSIBILITIES

Empowering patients and families to act as their own advocates requires that they have a clear understanding of their **rights and responsibilities**. These should be given (in print form) and/or presented (audio/video) to patients and families on admission, or as soon as possible.

- **Rights** should include competent, non-discriminatory medical care that respects privacy and allows participation in decisions about care and the right to refuse care. Patients and families should have clear, understandable explanations of treatments, options, and conditions, including outcomes. They should be apprised of transfers, changes in care plan, and advance directives. They should have access to medical records information about charges.
- **Responsibilities** should include providing honest and thorough information about health issues and medical history. Patients and families should ask for clarification if they don't understand information that is provided to them, and they should follow the plan of care that is outlined or explain why that is not possible. They should treat staff and other patients with respect.

> **Review Video: Patient Advocacy**
> Visit mometrix.com/academy and enter code: 202160

Patient Preparation

Introduction and Patient Identification

INITIATING PATIENT CONTACT

When initiating patient contact prior to conducting specimen collection, the following procedures should be followed:

1. Knock on the door before entering the patient's room, slowly open the door, and ask if you may enter.
2. Look for signs on the door indicating special precautions that must be taken (e.g., protective clothing needed).
3. Identify your name and reason for entering the room.
4. If a physician or member of the clergy is in the room, it may still be appropriate to explain who you are and proceed to do the draw if the draw is STAT.
5. If the patient is verbal, inquire about any issues (e.g., a history of fainting during venipuncture) or preferences (e.g., having family remain in the room vs. asking them to leave, telling the patient when the needle is about to be inserted vs. not telling them) they might have for the procedure.

IDENTIFYING THE PATIENT

The first step in any blood draw or laboratory procedure for inpatients and outpatients should be to properly **identify the patient**, using at least two forms of identification. Alert and responsive patients (or parents of a minor) may be asked to give their names and birthdates.

- Introduce yourself to the patient and explain your purpose.
- Check the ID band against information provided by the patient/caregiver/parent.
- Match specimen labeling to information on the ID band and label immediately with barcode labeler or permanent ink.
- Check ankles for an ID band if it is missing from wrists.
- Consider only the ID bands that are actually on the patient to be valid (not on bedside stand/bed) except in special circumstances (severe burns of extremities). Verify ID with nurse in these cases.
- If an armband is missing, procure an armband and secure it on the patient before the procedure.
- Ask outpatients for a picture ID and verify the name and birthdate verbally if possible.
- For emergent situations (unconscious patient in ED), check "Jane/John Doe" ID per protocol.
- For call reports, verify the patient's name, birthdate, and ID number.

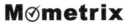

COMMUNICATING WITH A PATIENT

Prior to collecting a sample, it is important to make introductions to the patient, check the patient's identification, often through asking name and birthdate and checking wristband, and explain the purpose of the visit ("My name is John Doe, and I'm going to draw blood for the thyroid tests that your physician has ordered"). The phlebotomist should make a point of explaining actions ("I'm going to take a look at the veins in your arms") and should ask if the patient has a preference ("Where do you prefer to have blood drawn?") if possible. If patients, especially young children, are quite nervous or frightened, chatting with them briefly may help to distract them. The phlebotomist should remain professional and confident throughout the procedure and avoid making statements that may not be true (e.g., "You will barely feel this") because this violates the trust between the patient and phlebotomist.

PATIENT INTERVIEW

Interviewing strategies and techniques include:

- Establishing rapport with the patient: Take time to make introductions and talk for a moment, especially if the patient appears anxious.
- Positioning within the patient's field of vision: Position yourself face-to-face with the patient so that the patient does not have to look up or down during the interview.
- Avoiding medical jargon: Ask questions and respond in language that the patient is familiar with, and explain any unclear terms used.
- Ensuring patient privacy/confidentiality: Be alert to the surroundings and make sure that questions and the patient's responses remain confidential and cannot be overheard.
- Observing body language: Note nonverbal communication (eye contact, gestures, position, expressions, proxemics) for clues about the patient's emotional state and feelings.
- Asking open-ended questions: Avoid questions that can be answered with a simple "yes" or "no" as much as possible.
- Allowing patient time to respond: Do not look at a watch, fidget, or appear to be in a hurry.
- Practicing active listening: Make eye contact, nod, respond, and pay attention when the patient speaks.
- Respecting cultural differences: Avoid judgmental attitudes or comments.

Laboratory Orders

WRITTEN ORDERS FOR TESTS

Written and signed orders must be received for all tests, so telephone orders or verbal orders (such as in emergency situations) must be followed by a signed written order, which can be delivered, mailed, or electronically submitted to the laboratory. Tests may be ordered by the physician, the advanced practice nurse (such as a nurse practitioner), or the physician's assistant caring for the patient. The ordering healthcare provider must document in the patient's record the intention of having the test performed and the medical necessity for the test. Written orders should contain the date ordered, the time the test should be carried out, and the diagnostic code (ICD-10-CM) for each test ordered. The order should be appropriate for the diagnostic code, or CMS and insurance companies may not reimburse for the cost of the test.

ADD-ON REQUESTS

Add-on requests are tests ordered on the same sample after the original laboratory test is completed. Add-on requests, like all laboratory orders, must be received in writing—paper or electronic. The add-on requests may be part of the original order, indicating that if a test result is abnormal, then one or more additional tests should be carried out. The add-on test may also be ordered once the original test results are received. Add-on requests should indicate the sample that the add-on applies to. Some considerations include:

- Length of time the specimens are saved
- Storage: Refrigerated, room temperature, or frozen
- Specimen viability
- Adequacy of sample

For example, if a hematology sample is kept at room temperature, then some tests, such as CBC, can be carried out within 24 hours of collection time. Some tests (such as the reticulocyte count) can be carried out within 24 hours if the sample is refrigerated. Other tests must be conducted within 1–12 hours of collection time, depending on the type of specimen. Some add-on tests—including glucose, potassium, and bilirubin—should be avoided because the results may be inaccurate.

REQUISITION FORM

The requisition form is the form for entering the tests a patient is having, and the requisition then becomes part of the patient's permanent record. Requisition forms may be filled out manually or electronically. Electronic requisitions often automatically print out the labels with barcodes that will be affixed to the collection tubes. Required elements for a requisition form include the following:

- Name of ordering healthcare provider
- Patient's full name
- Patient's ID number (patient number if an inpatient)
- Room number if inpatient
- Patient's birthdate
- Test to be performed
- Test priorities
- Date and specific directions for test (e.g., "STAT" or "fasting")
- Billing information and codes as needed
- Allergies or any special precautions (e.g., "latex allergy" or "sensitive to adhesive")

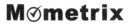

The laboratory professional should carefully check the requisition to make sure it is complete; verify the patient's identification before proceeding with sample collections; ensure any test requirements, such as "fasting," have been met; verify the date; and determine the priorities for collection.

PATIENT REGISTRATION AND TEST ORDER VERIFICATION

Patient registration requires obtaining information about the patient and entering that information into the records, which are usually in an internal database. The information required includes:

- The patient's name, address, Social Security number, birth date, telephone number, and email address (optional), and the name and telephone number of an emergency contact.
- Information about the responsible party. For example, if the patient is a child, the responsible party is generally a parent.
- Information about the policyholder's insurance, both primary and secondary. For example, patients on Medicare provide information about their Medicare coverage as well as any supplementary insurance.

Test order verification requires checking the laboratory order to ensure that it is correctly written, signed, and includes the ICD-10-CM diagnostic code for each order, and that each order is appropriate for the diagnosis. For Medicare/Medicaid, verification includes determining whether the test is covered, and within the appropriate time frame if it is a repeat test. Some tests may require preauthorization from insurance companies. The laboratory directory may be accessed to determine requirements for testing, such as minimum volume.

SAMPLE REGISTRATION

Sample registration begins with patient registration, which enters identifying information about the patient into the system. If an electronic laboratory information system (LIS) is in use, then labels and barcodes for specimen tubes are generated during patient registration. When the specimen is brought to the laboratory for processing, the sample is registered as part of the existing patient registration by retrieving the patient's file, based on the ID number assigned during initial information intake. If an LIS is not in use and laboratory records are done manually, labels and barcodes may be generated on arrival at the lab. The sample is assigned a number, and the time of the collection, arrival time, and type of tube and additive are all noted. The location of the sample is tracked, with the record indicating exactly where the sample is placed, such as the shelf, container, row, and number in a refrigerator if the sample is stored.

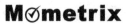

MINIMUM REQUIREMENTS FOR LABELING SPECIMENS

Laboratory specimens should always be labeled after collection with a label that is permanently attached (with adhesive). The tube or other container should never be labeled in advance, and permanent ink (generally black) should be used for any lettering:

- **Hand-written label**: A label must be hand-written with required information, which must include the patient's full name, ID number (temporary or permanent) if available, and date of birth, as well as the date and time of specimen collection and the phlebotomist's signature or initials.
- **Pre-printed label**: If a label is preprinted with the patient's name and other identifying information and/or a barcode, the phlebotomist must attach the label and write the date and time on the letter and sign with signature or initials.

Any special considerations, such as "fasting," should be noted on the label as well. Before the phlebotomist leaves the patient's side, the phlebotomist should compare the label on the specimen to the patient's ID bracelet or record and the laboratory requisition to ensure they all match. Once labeled, the specimen should be placed in a biohazard bag or container for transport.

LABORATORY RESULTS

Information that must be included on the laboratory results includes the name, address, and contact information for the lab; the patient's name, birthdate, gender, and ID number (if one is assigned); and the name of the requesting provider. The results must include the date and time the specimen was collected and the date and time each test result was verified. The tests should be listed along with the value, units, and reference ranges, with some indication of abnormal values, such as high (H), low (L), abnormal (A), critical high (CH), or critical low (CL). The lab results should be separated by type, such as chemistry panels and hematology panels. Laboratory results may be **distributed to ordering providers** in a number of different ways:

- **Paper**: Results may be delivered by courier, placed in the physician's hospital mailbox, or mailed.
- **Telephone**: Results may be transmitted by phone even when a paper or other type of report is given to ensure that the ordering provider receives the information in a timely manner, especially when there are abnormal results.
- **Messaging/email/electronic**: Results must be delivered over secure lines so that confidentiality is not compromised. Reports may be sent automatically. If patients can access through a patient portal, the ordering provider may need to access the report first and indicate that it can be released to the patient, depending on how the system is set up.

Cardiovascular System

CARDIOVASCULAR SYSTEM

LAYERS OF THE HEART

Three layers of tissue form the heart wall. The outer layer of the heart wall is the epicardium, the middle layer is the myocardium, and the inner layer is the endocardium:

- **Epicardium**: The membrane that covers the outside of the heart.
- **Myocardium**: The muscular wall of the heart (the thickest of the three layers of the heart wall) that lies between the inner layer (endocardium) and the outer layer (epicardium).
- **Endocardium**: The membrane lining the inside surface of the heart.

HEART CHAMBERS AND VALVES

There are four chambers of the heart. They have valves separating them, regulating a one-way flow of blood between the chambers.

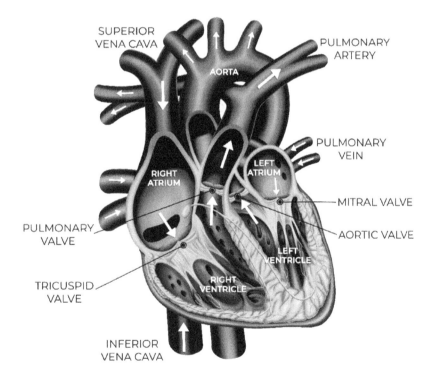

CARDIAC CYCLE

The cardiac cycle consists of ventricular diastole and ventricular systole.

- During **ventricular diastole**, the ventricles relax and the atria contract. Atrial contraction is regulated by the sinoatrial (SA) node, known as the pacemaker of the heart. The semilunar valves close (causing the "dub" sound), and the atrioventricular valves open, allowing the ventricles to fill.
- During **ventricular systole**, the ventricles contract, which is regulated by the atrioventricular (AV) node. The semilunar valves (the pulmonic valve and the aortic valve) open, allowing the ventricular contraction to pump blood to the lungs and to the periphery. The atrioventricular valve closes (causing the "lub" sound) to prevent backflow of blood from the ventricles into the atria.

37

ORIGIN OF HEART SOUNDS

A single heartbeat lasts about one second and consists of a two-part pumping action. As blood collects in both atria (the upper chambers of the heart), the SA node (the heart's natural pacemaker) sends an electrical signal that causes atrial contraction. This contraction forces blood through the mitral and tricuspid valves into the resting ventricles (the lower chambers). This is the longer part of the two-part pumping phase, and it is termed *diastole*. The pumping phase's second part begins after the ventricles have filled with blood. The electrical impulses from the SA node reach the AV node and then travel to the ventricles, signaling them to contract. This phase is called *systole*. During ventricular contraction, the mitral and tricuspid valves close tightly to prevent the backflow of blood, but the aortic and pulmonary valves are forced open. Blood ejected from the right ventricle travels to the lungs to get oxygenated. Oxygen-rich blood leaves the left ventricle to travel to all other areas of the body. The ventricles relax, and the pulmonary and aortic valves close after blood enters the aorta and pulmonary artery. The lower pressure in the ventricles causes the tricuspid and mitral valves to open, and the cycle begins again. This system of contractions is repeated, increasing during times of exertion and decreasing while at rest.

ELECTRICAL CONDUCTION SYSTEM

The heart beats (contracts) as a result of **electrical impulses** from the heart muscle (the myocardium). The electrical impulse starts in the **sinoatrial node (SA node)**, which is located in the top of the right atrium. Sometimes the SA node is referred to as the heart's "natural pacemaker." When the SA node releases the electrical signal, the atria contract. The signal is then passed through the **atrioventricular (AV) node**. After checking the signal, the AV node sends it through ventricular muscle fibers, causing them to contract. The SA node sends electrical impulses at a certain rate, but the heart rate may still change depending on physical demands, stress, or hormonal factors.

ECG TRACING OF CARDIAC CYCLE

ECG tracing of a cardiac cycle is as follows:

- **P wave** represents the atrial depolarization.
- **QRS complex** represents the ventricular depolarization.
- **T wave** represents the ventricular repolarization.

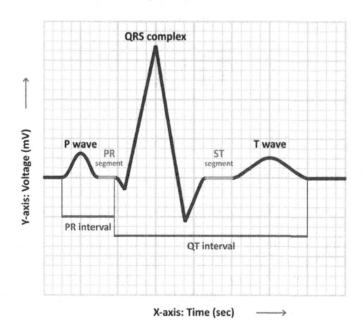

BLOOD VESSELS

The types of blood vessels are described below:

- **Arteries**: Blood vessels that carry blood away from the heart to the body (arteries do not have valves)
- **Veins**: Blood vessels that carry the blood from the body back to the heart (veins have valves)
- **Capillaries**: One-cell-thick blood vessels between arteries and veins that distribute oxygen-rich blood to the body
- **Venules**: The smallest veins
- **Arterioles**: The smallest arteries

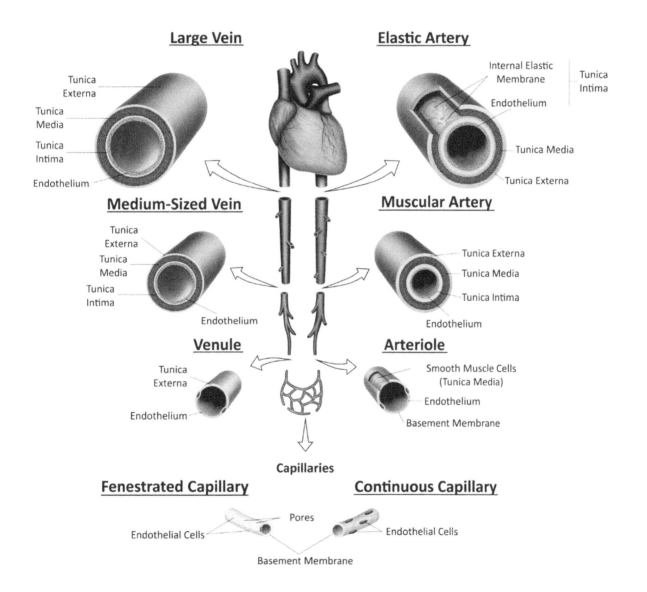

WALLS OF ARTERIES

The wall of an artery consists of three distinct layers of tunics:

- **Tunica intima**: Composed of simple, squamous epithelium called endothelium. Rests on a connective tissue membrane that is rich in elastic and collagenous fibers.
- **Tunica media**: Makes up the bulk of the arterial wall. Includes smooth muscle fibers, which encircle the tube, and a thick layer of elastic connective tissue.
- **Tunica adventitia** (tunica externa): Consists chiefly of connective tissue with irregularly arranged elastic and collagenous fibers. This layer attaches the artery to the surrounding tissues. Also contains minute vessels (vasa vasorum—vessels of vessels) that give rise to capillaries and provide blood to the more external cells of the artery wall.

Smooth muscles in the walls of arteries and arterioles are innervated by the sympathetic branches of the autonomic nervous system. The tunica media and the tunica adventitia are much thicker in arteries.

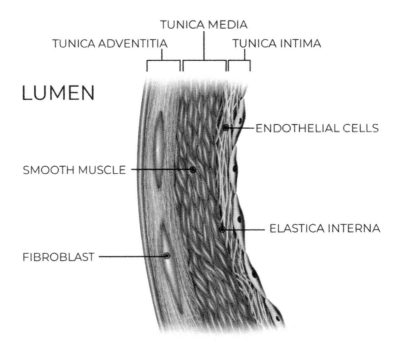

WALLS OF VEINS AND CAPILLARIES

Veins have the same three layers as arteries, but the middle layer is much thinner, so the walls are less muscular and less elastic, and the inner diameter is greater. Some veins, especially those in the arms and legs, contain flaplike valves to help prevent backflow. Veins can also serve as blood reservoirs during times of blood loss, constricting to move more blood to the heart.

Capillaries, extensions of the endothelium, are composed of a thin permeable layer of squamous epithelium through which substances in the blood are exchanged for those in tissue.

VEINS OF THE LOWER EXTREMITY

The great saphenous, popliteal, femoral, and lesser saphenous veins are the major **veins** returning blood to the heart from the lower extremities:

- **Great saphenous**: Runs the entire length of the lower extremity and is the longest vein in the body.
- **Popliteal**: Runs deep behind the knee.
- **Femoral**: Runs deep in the upper part of the leg.
- **Lesser saphenous**: Runs lateral to the ankle, up the leg, and deep behind the knee.

ARTERIES OF THE UPPER EXTREMITIES

The arteries of the upper extremities are described below:

- **Internal thoracic**: Descends posteriorly to the clavicle's sternal end and enters the thorax
- **Thyrocervical trunk**: Ascends and gives off four different branches, including the transverse and ascending cervical arteries and the suprascapular artery
- **Suprascapular**: Travels inferolaterally, follows the clavicle in a parallel manner, then goes posteriorly to the scapula
- **Subscapular**: Descends along subscapularis muscle's lateral border to the inferior angle of the scapula
- **Thoracodorsal**: Accompanies the nerve of the same name to the latissimus dorsi muscle
- **Deep brachial**: Accompanies the radial nerve as they both pass through the humeral radial groove, then it anastomoses around the elbow joint
- **Ulnar collateral**: Anastomoses around the elbow joint

BLOOD MOVEMENT IN THE CIRCULATORY SYSTEM

The blood flowing through the arterial system is pushed by the pressure built up by the contractions of the heart. The blood flowing through the veins relies on skeletal muscle movement to keep the valves located in the veins opening and closing, to keep blood moving toward the heart and not backward through the system.

> **Review Video: Cardiovascular System**
> Visit mometrix.com/academy and enter code: 376581
>
> **Review Video: Heart Blood Flow**
> Visit mometrix.com/academy and enter code: 783139

Vascular System Functions

The main functions of the vascular system include the following:

- **Transports** cellular and chemical materials
  - Gases—Oxygen is shuttled to the cells from the lungs, and carbon dioxide (a waste product) is transported to the lungs from the cells.
  - Nutrients—In addition to oxygen, other nutrients, like glucose, are transported via the circulatory system. Glucose is shuttled to the liver immediately after digestion. Glucose is used to make ATP (cellular energy), and the liver functions to maintain a stable blood glucose level.
  - Cellular waste—Waste products from digestion, such as ammonia (produced from protein digestion), are transported to the liver to be converted to a less toxic substance, urea, which then moves on to the kidneys and is eventually excreted in the urine.
  - Hormones—The vascular system transports numerous hormones that function to maintain constant internal conditions.
- Contains infection-fighting cells
- Helps stabilize body fluid pH and ionic concentration
- Transports **heat** to help maintain body temperature

Blood and Blood Components

Blood has numerous functions—gas transport, hemostasis, defense against disease—all of which are brought about by its various components:

- **Red blood cells**: Oxygen transport and gas exchange
- **Blood platelets and coagulation factors**: Coagulation and hemostasis
- **Vitamin K**: Essential cofactor in normal hepatic synthesis of some clotting factors
- **Plasmin**: Lyses fibrin and fibrinogen
- **Antithrombin III**: Inhibits IXa, Xa, XIa, XIIa
- **Complement**: Defense against pyogenic bacteria, activation of phagocytes, clearing of immune complexes, and lytic attack on cell membranes
- **Lymphocytes**: Adaptive immune response—killing of specific microbes
- **Monocytes**: Respond to necrotic cell material by migrating to tissues and differentiating into macrophages
- **Neutrophils**: Phagocytosis of microbes
- **Eosinophils**: Phagocytosis, defense against helminthic parasites, allergic reactions
- **Basophils**: Allergic reactions

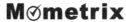

WHOLE BLOOD, PLASMA, AND SERUM

Whole blood is blood as it is withdrawn from the body. It contains the following:

- Plasma, which includes clotting factors
- Erythrocytes (red blood cells)
- Leukocytes (white blood cells), which include:
  - Monocytes
  - Lymphocytes
  - Neutrophils
  - Basophils
  - Eosinophils
- Thrombocytes (platelets)

Whole blood is rarely used for testing or administration but is separated into components.

Plasma is the liquid portion of the blood that is free of cells because the erythrocytes, leukocytes, and thrombocytes have been removed. It still contains clotting factors, such as fibrinogen, because it has been treated with an anticoagulant, such as sodium citrate.

Serum, on the other hand, is the liquid portion of blood that is also cell-free but has been allowed to clot and is then spun to separate and remove the clot so that it is also free of clotting factors. Serum is more often used for testing than plasma because serum contains more antigens and can be used for a wider variety of tests. Additionally, anticoagulants found in plasma may interfere with some tests.

RED BLOOD CELLS, WHITE BLOOD CELLS, AND PLATELETS

Blood cells are produced in the bone marrow. Blood is a viscous dark red fluid composed of cells, gases, and plasma (55%). Blood components include:

- **Erythrocytes** (red blood cells): Red blood cells carry hemoglobin, which transports oxygen. If red blood cell count is low (such as from blood loss) or oxygen-carrying capacity is impaired (such as with anemia), the patient may experience hypoxemia (low oxygen). The life cycle is normally 120 days.
- **Leukocytes** (white blood cells): WBCs defend the body against invading organisms (viruses, bacteria, fungi, and parasites) in the bloodstream and tissues, and they respond to allergies. WBCs include lymphocytes (B, T, natural killer cells, and null cells), monocytes, eosinophils, basophils, and neutrophils.
- **Thrombocytes** (platelets): Platelets release clotting factors and have an active role in forming blood clots.
- **Plasma** (55% of blood): Plasma carries water, proteins, electrolytes, lipids (fats), blood cells, and glucose, as well as clotting factors.

The primary **blood types** are A, B, AB, and O. Blood is either Rh– or Rh+, and patients must receive transfusions of blood that are type- and Rh-compatible.

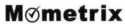

OXYGENATION AND OXIDATION OF HEMOGLOBIN

Oxygenation is the loose, reversible binding of hemoglobin (Hgb) with O_2 molecules, forming oxyhemoglobin. Hgb oxygenation is the principal method of O_2 uptake from the lungs into the RBCs for transport to the tissues. Each Hgb molecule has the capacity to bind four O_2 molecules since there are four heme molecules in each Hgb. The O_2 binds loosely with the coordination bonds of the iron atom in the heme and not the two positive bonds of the iron. Iron is not oxidized, and oxygen can be carried to the tissues in the molecular form rather than the ionic form.

Oxidation of Hgb involves the conversion of the functional ferrous (Fe^{2+}) heme iron to the non-functional ferric (Fe^{3+}) form. This is called methemoglobin. This oxidized form of Hgb can't bind or transport oxygen. Oxidation of Hgb may occur due to exposure to toxic chemicals such as nitrites, aniline dyes, and oxidative drugs.

IMMUNOGLOBULIN

Immunoglobulins are proteins created by plasma that attach to foreign substances (bacteria, viruses, etc.), which neutralizes them and ultimately destroys them. The **types of immunoglobulins** and their functions are explained below:

- **IgA**: Can be located in secretions and prevents viral and bacterial attachment to membranes
- **IgD**: Can be located on B cells and signals for their activation against foreign substances
- **IgE**: The main mediator of mast cells with an allergen exposure
- **IgG**: Primarily found in secondary responses, can cross the placenta, and destroys viruses/bacteria
- **IgM**: Primarily found in first response, located on B cells

ANEMIA

Anemia refers to any condition where there is reduced oxygen-carrying capacity due to a fall in hemoglobin concentration with resultant tissue hypoxia. It is defined as Hgb <13.5 g/dL in males, <11.5 g/dL in females, <15 g/dL in newborns to three-month-old infants, and <11 g/dL from three months to puberty. Anemia results when compensatory mechanisms fail to restore oxygen levels to meet tissue demands. The following compensatory mechanisms can be seen:

- Arteriolar dilatation
- Increased cardiac output
- Increased anaerobic metabolism
- Increased Hgb dissociation
- Increased erythropoietin output
- Internal redistribution of blood flow

If these compensatory mechanisms are adequate, oxygen levels are restored. If not, anemia ensues, with cardiac effects, poor exercise tolerance, lethargy, pallor, headaches, angina on effort, and claudication.

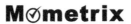

Medical Terminology

ORIGIN OF MEDICAL TERMINOLOGY

Most medical terms derive from Greek or Latin, but there are a few English, French, and German terms. If a Greek or Latin word is broken down into its root, prefix, and suffix, one can understand unfamiliar terminology. To avoid awkward pronunciation when there is no vowel between the root word and suffix, add an *-o-* to the combining form. For instance, add the suffix *-metry* (meaning the measure of) to the root word for eye (*opt*) along with the combining *-o-* to make the word *optometry*. Examples of English terminology include: Epstein-Barr virus, HIV-positive, 100-mL sample, oxygen-dependent, and self-image. As seen in these examples, English words use a hyphen instead of a joining vowel. An example of French terminology is *grand mal* (big sickness) for epileptic seizures. An example of German terminology is *mittelschmerz* (middle pain) for the discomfort of ovulation. French and German do not have convenient combining forms, so they must be memorized.

PREFIX, SUFFIX, AND ROOT

Medical terms have three parts:

- **Prefix**: Before the root, modifies the meaning
- **Suffix**: After the root, modifies the meaning
- **Root**: Contains the basic meaning

Examples:

- *Menorrhagia* is excessive bleeding during menstruation. The root is *meno*, meaning menstruation. The suffix is *-rrhagia*, meaning a flow that bursts forth.
- *Rhinoplasty* is a nose job. The root is *rhino*, meaning nose. The suffix is *-plasty*, meaning reconstructive surgery.
- *Antecubitum* is the bend of the arm where the nurse draws blood. The root is *cubitum*, meaning elbow. The prefix is *ante-*, meaning forward or before.

PREFIXES

Prefix	Meaning	Example
ab-	from, not here, off the norm	abnormal
ad-	to, in the direction of	adduct
ante-	prior to, in front of, previously	antecedent
anti-	hostile to, against, contradictory	antisocial
be-	make, aligned with, greatly	benign
bi-	two, occurring twice	bicycle
de-	away, versus, reduce	deduct
dia-	transverse, across	diameter
dis-	contradictory, disparate, away	disjointed
en-	create, put in or on, surround	engulf
syn-	by means of, together, same	synthesis
trans-	across, far away, go through	transvaginal
ultra-	extreme, beyond in space	ultrasound
un-	opposing, antithetical, not	uncooperative

The following is a list of additional **medical terminology prefixes**:

Prefix	Meaning	Prefix	Meaning
a-	without	*multi-*	numerous
an-	without	*neo-*	new
bin-	two	*nulli-*	none
brady-	slow	*pan-*	total
dys-	difficult	*para-*	beyond
endo-	within	*per-*	through
epi-	over	*peri-*	surrounding
eu-	normal	*poly-*	many
ex-	outward	*post-*	after
exo-	outward	*pre-*	before
hemi-	half	*pro-*	before
hyper	excessive	*sub-*	below
hypo-	deficient	*supra-*	superior
inter-	between	*sym-*	join
intra-	within	*tachy-*	rapid
meta-	change	*tetra-*	four
micro-	minute, tiny	*uni-*	one

SUFFIXES

Suffix	Meaning	Example
-fication/-ation	manner or process	classification
-gram	written down or illustrated	cardiogram
-graph	a machine or instrument that records data	cardiograph
-graphy	the process of recording of data	cardiography
-ics	science or skill of	synthetics
-itis	red, inflamed, swollen	bursitis
-meter	means of measure	thermometer
-metry	action of measuring	telemetry
-ology/-ogy	the study of	biology
-phore	bearer or maker	semaphore
-phobia	intense, irrational fear	arachnophobia
-scope	instrument used for visualizing data	microscope
-scopy	the process of visualizing or examining	bronchoscopy

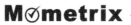

The following is a list of additional **medical terminology suffixes**:

Suffix	Meaning
-ac	pertaining to
-ad	toward
-al	pertaining to
-algia	pain
-apheresis	removal
-ar	pertaining to
-ary	pertaining to
-asthenia	weakness
-atresia	occlusion, closure
-capnia	carbon dioxide
-cele	hernia
-centesis	surgical puncture
-clasia	break
-clasis	break
-coccus	berry-like bacteria
-crit	separate
-cyte	cell
-desis	fusion
-drome	run
-eal	pertaining to
-ectasis	expansion
-ectomy	removal
-emia	blood dysfunction
-esis	condition
-gen	agent that causes
-genesis	cause
-genic	pertaining to
-ia	disease condition
-ial	pertaining to
-iasis	condition
-iatrist	physician
-iatry	specialty
-ician	a person skilled in
-ictal	attack
-ior	pertaining to
-ism	condition of
-lysis	separating
-malacia	softening
-megaly	increasing in size
-odynia	pain
-oid	resembling
-ologist	person that practices

Suffix	Meaning
-oma	tumor
-opia	vision
-opsy	view of
-orrhagia	blood flowing profusely
-orrhaphy	repairing
-orrhea	flow
-orrhexis	break
-osis	condition
-ostomy	to make an opening
-otomy	cut into
-ous	pertaining to
-oxia	oxygen
-paresis	partial paralysis
-pathy	disease
-penia	decrease in number
-pepsia	digestion
-pexy	suspension
-phagia	swallowing, eating
-phonia	sound, voice
-physis	growth
-plasia	development
-plasm	a growth
-plasty	repair by surgery
-plegia	paralysis
-pnea	breathing
-poiesis	formation
-ptosis	sagging
-salpinx	fallopian tube
-sarcoma	malignant tumor
-schisis	crack
-sclerosis	hardening
-sis	condition of
-spasm	abnormal muscle firing
-stasis	standing
-stenosis	narrowing
-thorax	chest
-tocia	labor, birth
-tome	cutting device
-tripsy	surgical crushing
-trophy	develop
-uria	urine

WORD ROOTS

The following is a list of common **medical terminology word roots**:

Root Word	Meaning	Root Word	Meaning
abdomin/o	abdomen	chrom/o	color
acou/o	hearing	clavic/o	clavicle
acr/o	height/extremities	col/o	colon
aden/o	gland	colp/o	vagina
adren/o	adrenal gland	core/o	pupil
alveol/o	alveolus	corne/o	cornea
amni/o	amnion	coron/o	heart
andro/o	male	cortic/o	cortex
angi/o	vessel	cor/o	pupil
ankyl/o	stiff	cost/o	rib
anter/o	frontal	crani/o	cranium
an/o	anus	cry/o	cold
aponeur/o	aponeurosis	cutane/o	skin
appendic/o	appendix	cyan/o	blue
arche/o	beginning	cyes/i	pregnancy
arteri/o	artery	cyst/o	bladder
athero/o	fatty plaque	cyt/o	cell
atri/o	atrium	dacry/o	tear
auri/o	ear	derm/o	skin
aut/o	self	diaphragmat/o	diaphragm
azot/o	nitrogen	dipl/o	double
bacteri/o	bacteria	dips/o	thirst
balan/o	glans penis	disk/o	disk
bi/o	life	dist/o	distal
blast/o	developing cell	diverticul/o	diverticulum
blephar/o	eyelid	dors/o	back
bronchi/o	bronchus	duoden/o	duodenum
burs/o	bursa	dur/o	dura
calc/i	calcium	ech/o	sound
carcin/o	cancer	electr/o	electricity
cardi/o	heart	embry/o	embryo
carp/o	carpals	encephal/o	brain
caud/o	tail	endocrin/o	endocrine
cec/o	cecum	enter/o	intestine
celi/o	abdomen	epididym/o	epididymis
cephal/o	head	epiglott/o	epiglottis
cerebell/o	cerebellum	episi/o	vulva
cerebr/o	cerebrum	erythr/o	red
cervic/o	cervix	esophag/o	esophagus
cheil/o	lip	esthesi/o	sensation
cholangi/o	bile duct	eti/o	cause of disease
chol/e	gall	femor/o	femur
chondr/o	cartilage	feti/o	fetus
chori/o	chorion	fibr/o	fibrous tissue

48

Root Word	Meaning	Root Word	Meaning
fibul/o	fibula	mandibul/o	mandible
gangli/o	ganglion	mast/o	breast
gastr/o	stomach	maxill/o	maxilla
gingiv/o	gum	meat/o	opening
glomerul/o	glomerulus	melan/o	dark, black
gloss/o	tongue	mening/o	meninges
glyc/o	sugar	menisc/o	meniscus
gnos/o	knowledge	men/o	menstruation
gravid/o	pregnancy	ment/o	mind
gyn/o	woman	metri/o	uterus
hem/o	blood	mon/o	one
hepat/o	liver	muc/o	mucus
herni/o	hernia	myc/o	fungus
heter/o	other	myel/o	spinal cord
hidr/o	sweat	myelon/o	bone marrow
hist/o	tissue	myos/o	muscle
humer/o	humerus	nas/o	nose
hydr/o	water	nat/o	birth
hymen/o	hymen	necr/o	death
hyster/o	uterus	nephr/o	kidney
ile/o	ileum	neur/o	nerve
ili/o	ilium	noct/i	night
infer/o	inferior	ocul/o	eye
irid/o	iris	olig/o	few
ischi/o	ischium	omphal/o	navel
ischo/o	blockage	onc/o	tumor
jejun/o	jejunum	onych/o	nail
kal/i	potassium	oophor/o	ovary
kary/o	nucleus	ophthalm/o	eye
kerat/o	hard	opt/o	vision
kinesi/o	motion	orch/o	testicle
kyph/o	hump	organ/o	organ
lacrim/o	tear duct	or/o	mouth
lact/o	milk	orth/o	straight
lamin/o	lamina	oste/o	bone
lapar/o	abdomen	ot/o	ear
laryng/o	larynx	ox/i	oxygen
later/o	lateral	pachy/o	thick
lei/o	smooth	palat/o	palate
leuk/o	white	pancreat/o	pancreas
lingu/o	tongue	parathyroid/o	parathyroid gland
lip/o	fat	par/o	labor
lith/o	stone	patell/o	patella
lord/o	flexed forward	path/o	disease
lumb/o	lumbar	pelv/i	pelvis
lymph/o	lymph	perine/o	peritoneum
mamm/o	breast	petr/o	stone

Root Word	Meaning	Root Word	Meaning
phalang/o	pharynx	sphygm/o	pulse
phas/o	speech	spir/o	breathe
phleb/o	vein	splen/o	spleen
phot/o	light	spondyl/o	vertebra
phren/o	mind	staped/o	stapes
plasm/o	plasma	staphyl/o	clusters
pleur/o	pleura	stern/o	sternum
pneum/o	lung	steth/o	chest
poli/o	gray matter	stomat/o	mouth
polyp/o	small growth	strept/o	chain-like
poster/o	posterior	super/o	superior
prim/i	first	synovi/o	synovia
proct/o	rectum	tars/o	tarsal
prostat/o	prostate gland	ten/o	tendon
proxim/o	proximal	test/o	testicle
pseud/o	fake	therm/o	heat
psych/o	mind	thorac/o	thorax
pub/o	pubis	thromb/o	clot
puerper/o	childbirth	thym/o	thymus
pulmon/o	lung	thyr/o	thyroid gland
pupill/o	pupil	tibi/o	tibia
pyel/o	renal pelvis	tom/o	cut
pylor/o	pylorus	tonsil/o	tonsils
py/o	pus	toxic/o	poison
quadr/i	four	trachel/o	trachea
rachi/o	spinal	trich/o	hair
radic/o	nerve	tympan/o	eardrum
radi/o	radius	uln/o	ulna
rect/o	rectum	ungu/o	nail
ren/o	kidney	ureter/o	ureter
retin/o	retina	urethr/o	urethra
rhabd/o	striated	ur/o	urine
rhin/o	nose	uter/o	uterus
rhytid/o	wrinkles	uvul/o	uvula
rhiz/o	root, nerve	vagin/o	vagina
salping/o	tube	valv/o	valve
sacr/o	sacrum	vas/o	vessel
scapul/o	scapula	ven/o	vein
scler/o	sclera	ventricul/o	ventricle
scoli/o	curved	ventro/o	frontal
seb/o	sebum	vertebr/o	vertebra
sept/o	septum	vesic/o	bladder
sial/o	saliva	vesicul/o	seminal vesicles
sinus/o	sinus	viscer/o	internal organs
somat/o	body	vulv/o	vulva
son/o	sound	xanth/o	yellow
spermat/o	sperm	xer/o	dry

STANDARDIZED TERMINOLOGY AND ABBREVIATIONS

Standardized terminology and abbreviations are vital for patient safety. Use abbreviations to save time and space *only when there is no potential for confusion over the meaning of the message.* Avoid Latin if there is an accepted English equivalent. The medical records manager decides acceptable terminology and forbidden abbreviations. If you are working in a small office and are in charge of medical records, use the list of safe terms from the American Society for Testing and Materials (ASTM) and the list of dangerous abbreviations from the Institute for Safe Medication Practices (ISMP). The Joint Commission also has a "Do Not Use" list for medical abbreviations and symbols that are included on the ISMP's more comprehensive list. Post them throughout the office. Use one type of units only. For example, do not use SI units (International System of Measurement) for the lab and Imperial units for the pharmacy without listing equivalencies. Adopt the US Postal Service database's two-letter abbreviations for states.

Health professionals use abbreviations to save time when charting or to be discreet when speaking around a patient. Abbreviations take these forms:

- *Brief form* means shortening a common term or difficult-to-pronounce term. For example, shortening *telephone* to *phone* or *Papanicolaou smear* to *Pap smear.*
- *Acronym* means making a word out of a phrase. For example: *LASER* stands for "light amplification by stimulated emission of radiation."
- *Initialism* means making a word from the first letters of words in a phrase, and pronouncing the series of letters. For example, *MRI* is used for "magnetic resonance imaging," and *HIV* is used for "human immunodeficiency virus."
- *Eponym* means naming a test or sign for its discoverer. For example: Coombs test, McBurney's sign.

MEDICAL ABBREVIATIONS AND ACRONYMS

Abbreviation or Acronym	Meaning
AIDS	acquired immunodeficiency syndrome
A.D.	right ear, auris dextra (on ISMP's list of error-prone abbreviations)
A.S.	left ear, auris sinistra (on ISMP's list of error-prone abbreviations)
A.U.	both ears, auris utraque (on ISMP's list of error-prone abbreviations)
O.D.	right eye, oculus dexter (on ISMP's list of error-prone abbreviations)
O.S.	left eye, oculus sinister (on ISMP's list of error-prone abbreviations)
O.U.	both eyes, oculus uterque (on ISMP's list of error-prone abbreviations)
CA	cancer or carcinoma
CBC and diff	complete blood count and differential
CHF	congestive heart failure
TAHBSO	complete hysterectomy; total abdominal hysterectomy, bilateral salpingo-oophorectomy
CABG	(pronounced "cabbage") coronary artery bypass graft
DNR	do not resuscitate; no codes should be called for this patient, and no heroic measures should be taken to revive patient if the patient stops breathing
DTR	deep tendon reflexes
D&C	dilation and curettage, used to cure uterine bleeding or for early abortion
ECG or EKG	electrocardiogram
ELISA	enzyme-linked immunosorbent assay, used to test for antibodies and antigens
FABERE	flexion abduction external rotation extension test, part of a physical to measure the patient's range of motion
HPI	history of present illness
LASER	light amplification by stimulated emission of radiation, a tool to carve tissue
P&A	percussion and auscultation, as in, "The lungs were clear to P&A."
PVH	persistent viral hepatitis
PND	postnasal drainage (can also mean paroxysmal nocturnal dyspnea in a sleep study)
simkin	simulation kinetics analysis
p.c.	*post cibum*, after meals
a.c.	*ante cibum*, before meals
h.s.	*hora somni*, bedtime

ADDITIONAL COMMON ABBREVIATIONS

Abbreviation	Meaning
ad lib	Freely or whenever desired
ANS	Autonomic nervous system
ant	Anterior
ASAP	As soon as possible
AV	Arteriovenous, atrioventricular
bid	Twice a day
BP	Blood pressure
bpm	Beats per minute
BUN	Blood urea nitrogen
Bx	Biopsy
C&S	Culture and sensitivity
Ca	Calcium
CC	Colony count
cc	Cubic centimeters
CEA	Carcinoembryonic antigen
Cl	Chloride
cm	Centimeters
CNS	Central nervous system
CPK	Creatine phosphokinase
CPR	Cardiopulmonary resuscitation
CSF	Cerebrospinal fluid
CV	Cardiovascular
CVP	Central venous pressure
D/C	Discharge
DW	Distilled water
Dx	Diagnosis
EBL	Estimated blood loss
e.m.p.	In the manner prescribed
ERT	Estrogen replacement therapy
ESR	Erythrocyte sedimentation rate
etiol	Etiology
FBS	Fasting blood sugar
Fe	Iron
FSH	Follicle-stimulating hormone
g	Grams
GERD	Gastroesophageal reflux disease
Grad.	Gradually
GTT	Glucose tolerance test

Abbreviation	Meaning
gtt	Drops
hr	Hour
H or hypo.	Hypodermic
HD	Hemodialysis
H&H	Hemoglobin and hematocrit
Hct	Hematocrit
Hg	Mercury
Hgb	Hemoglobin
HIV	Human immunodeficiency virus
H&P	History and physical
IM	Intramuscular
IV	Intravenous
K	Potassium
KCl	Potassium chloride
kg	Kilograms
KVO	Keep vein open
lab	Laboratory
meds	Medications
mEq	Milliequivalents
MS	Multiple sclerosis
Na	Sodium
NB	Newborn
neg	Negative
NPO	Nothing by mouth
OD	Daily
O_2	Oxygen
PCV	Packed cell volume
PM	Between noon and midnight
pos.	Positive
post-op	Postoperatively
PRBC	Packed red blood cells
p.r.n.	As needed
PSA	Prostate-specific antigen
PT	Prothrombin time
PT	Physical therapy
qd	Every day
qid	Four times a day
qod	Every other day
q4h	Every four hours
STAT	Immediately
tid	Three times a day

PLURALIZING MEDICAL TERMS

Most medical laboratory terms derive from Latin and Greek. Most Latinate terms originated from the Greek. The basic rules for pluralizing medical terms are as follows:

Rule	Example
-*a* changes to -*ata*	Stig*ma* to stigm*ata* Condylo*ma* to condylom*ata*
-*on* changes to -*a*	Criteri*on* to criteri*a* Phenomen*on* to phenomen*a*
-*s* changes to -*des*	Iri*s* to iri*des* Arthriti*s* to arthriti*des*
Feminine -*a* ending changes to -*ae*	Uln*a* to uln*ae* Conch*a* to conch*ae*
Masculine ending -*us* changes to -*i*	Radi*us* to radi*i* Muscul*us* to muscul*i*
Neuter ending -*um* changes to -*a*	Bacteri*um* to bacteri*a* Strat*um* to strat*a*
-*osis* changes to -*oses*	Diagn*osis* to diagn*oses* Anastom*osis* to anastom*oses*
-*x* changes to -*ces* or -*ges*	Phalan*x* to phalan*ges* Vari*x* to vari*ces*

MEDICAL AND SURGICAL SPECIALTIES

The suffix -*ology* means "study of," and the suffixes -*iatry* and -*iatrics* refer to "medical treatment." Add the body system root to obtain the name of the specialty:

Term	Meaning
Anesthesiology	Study of pain relief
Bariatrics	Treatment of obesity
Cardiology	Study of the heart
Dermatology	Study of the skin
Endocrinology	Study of the hormone system
Gastroenterology	Study of the digestive system
Geriatrics	Treatment of the elderly
Hematology	Study of the blood
Neurology	Study of the nervous system
Obstetrics	Treatment of pregnant women
Pediatrics	Treatment of children
Psychiatry	Treatment of the mind
Radiology	Study of radiation (for medical imaging)
Rheumatology	Study of rheumatoid diseases, like arthritis
Toxicology	Study of poisons
Urology	Study of the urinary system

REFERENCE SOURCES FOR MEDICAL TERMINOLOGY

Reliable **reference sources** to check correct spelling, and selection and use of medical terminology, are listed below:

- **Abbreviations**: Use safe terms and definitions from the American Society for Testing and Materials (ASTM). Obtain a list of dangerous abbreviations to be avoided from the Institute for Safe Medication Practices (ISMP).
- **Style guides**: Provide guidelines for format and presentation in documents. Use *American Medical Association Manual of Style: A Guide for Authors and Editors* for an overview.
- **Anatomy and physiology texts**: Contain essential information regarding body structure, functions of body parts, disease processes, and common health disorders. *Gray's Anatomy* is the classic.
- **Specialty texts**: When help is required with specialty transcriptions, try Sloane's *Medical Word Book*, Tessier's *Surgical Word Book*, and Pagana's *Laboratory and Diagnostic Tests*.
- **English dictionary**: Helps with spelling, definitions, and pronunciation. *Cambridge Dictionary of American English* is the standard.

CONVERSION CHART OF METRIC TO ENGLISH

	Metric	**English**
Distance	meter	3.3 feet
Mass	gram	0.0022 pounds
	kilogram	2.2 pounds
Volume	liter	1.06 quarts

ROMAN NUMERALS

The following **Roman numerals** have the values shown.

$$I = 1$$
$$V = 5$$
$$X = 10$$
$$L = 50$$
$$C = 100$$
$$D = 500$$
$$M = 1,000$$

MILITARY AND CIVILIAN TIME

Military	=	Civilian		Military	=	Civilian
0100	=	1:00 AM		1300	=	1:00 PM
0200	=	2:00 AM		1400	=	2:00 PM
0300	=	3:00 AM		1500	=	3:00 PM
0400	=	4:00 AM		1600	=	4:00 PM
0500	=	5:00 AM		1700	=	5:00 PM
0600	=	6:00 AM		1800	=	6:00 PM
0700	=	7:00 AM		1900	=	7:00 PM
0800	=	8:00 AM		2000	=	8:00 PM
0900	=	9:00 AM		2100	=	9:00 PM
1000	=	10:00 AM		2200	=	10:00 PM
1100	=	11:00 AM		2300	=	11:00 PM
1200	=	12 Noon		0000	=	12 Midnight

FORMULAS AND CONVERSIONS

Fahrenheit into Celsius

$$C = (F - 32) \times \frac{5}{9}$$

Celsius into Fahrenheit

$$F = \left(C \times \frac{9}{5}\right) + 32$$

Pounds into kilograms

$$\text{kilograms} = \text{pounds} \times 0.4536$$

Equation to determine percentage

$$(\text{amount} \div \text{total}) \times 100 = \text{percentage}$$

APPROXIMATING LITERS OF BLOOD IN NORMAL ADULTS

The average adult has 70 mL of blood per kilogram of weight. In the United States, a person's weight is usually recorded in pounds. The phlebotomist will need to convert the pounds into kilograms by using the conversion factor of 0.4536. The person's weight in kilograms is multiplied by 70, the average mL of blood per kilogram. Then divide that number by 1,000 to convert the mL into liters.

APPROXIMATING LITERS OF BLOOD IN INFANTS

The average infant has 100 mL of blood per kilogram of weight. If an infant's weight is given in pounds, it must be converted to kilograms using the conversion factor of 0.454. That number is then multiplied by 100, which is the average mL of blood per kilogram in an infant. Then divide that number by 1,000 to convert the mL into liters.

Routine Blood Collections

Blood Sample Collection Supplies and Equipment

EQUIPMENT FOR BLOOD COLLECTION

Equipment needed for blood collection includes:

- Phlebotomy cart or tray to hold equipment for easy access.
- PPE, including gloves: Latex gloves should be avoided, as many patients are allergic to latex, and powdered gloves pose a risk of sample contamination. Glove liners can be used for phlebotomists who are sensitive to gloves.
- Antiseptics: Isopropyl alcohol 70%, povidone iodine, and chlorhexidine gluconate are the most commonly used.
- Gauze pads and bandages: Cotton balls should not be used to apply pressure on the puncture site because they may adhere to the tissue and cause bleeding when removed.
- Vein-locating devices: Use if necessary and available.
- Tourniquet: Non-latex are preferable. Various sizes should be available, including extra-large for obese patients and pediatric sizes. They should be flat and about 1 inch in width. They may be disposable or reusable.
- Needles, syringes, tube holders, and evacuated collection tubes of various types, depending on the tests to be performed.
- Sharps container: These must be available to dispose of needles.

NEEDLE GAUGE AND SELECTION

The gauge of a needle is a number that is inversely correlated to the diameter of the internal space of the needle. The larger the needle gauge, the smaller the internal space of the needle, and vice versa. Since color-coding varies between manufacturers, be careful of relying on color to determine the gauge of a needle. When selecting a needle for venipuncture, there are several factors to consider, including the type of procedure, the condition and size of the patient's vein, and the equipment being used. The length of the needle used is determined by the depth of the vein. Keep in mind that the smaller the gauge, the larger the bore. The 21-gauge needle is the standard needle used for routine venipuncture.

NEEDLE SAFETY DEVICES

Needle safety devices protect the needle user's hand by having it remain behind the needle during use and by providing a barrier between the user's hand and the needle after use. Also, needle safety devices are operable with a one-handed technique and provide a permanent barrier around the contaminated needle. By activating the safety device after use, the needle cover (generally a plastic top) clicks over the needle into a permanent, locked position. The needle cannot be reused nor inadvertently become exposed after the safety device is locked into place.

BUTTERFLY NEEDLE

If a patient—such as a child, or an adult who is very thin with prominent veins—requires a low needle angle or depth for venipuncture, the best choice is a **winged infusion ("butterfly") set** that allows a very low angle (10–15°) for venipuncture, as the needle can be held almost parallel to the skin. Winged needles are also useful to access hand veins and the scalp veins of infants. The needle (usually 23-gauge, although 25-gauge may be used if vessels are extremely small) ranges from 0.5 to 0.75 inches in length, with 6–15 inches of tubing to which the syringe is attached. Vacutainers can also attach to the end of the tubing on which blood collection tubes can be inserted and directly draw a sample. For insertion, the flexible wings are grasped to guide the needle. A flash can be observed in the collection chamber of the butterfly, and then blood can be withdrawn using the syringe or pressure of the vacutainer.

Butterfly Needle Infusion Set

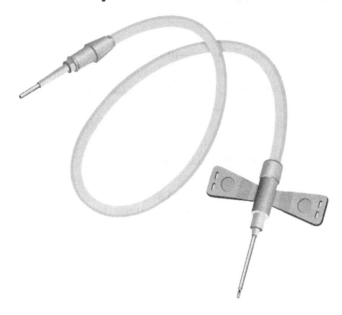

SYRINGE SYSTEM

In straightforward venipunctures, the syringe system may be used. A syringe is attached directly to the venipuncture needle, which contains a small hub in which a "flash" can be visualized when the vein is accessed. The syringe can pull back the required volume of blood and then distribute that blood into the appropriate blood tubes.

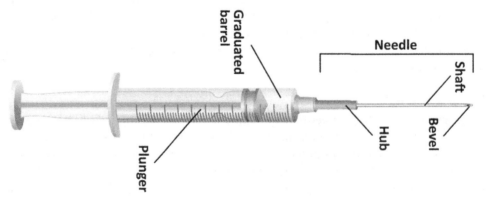

TOURNIQUET

A tourniquet is used to aid in the collection of a blood specimen. The tourniquet is tied in such a way that it can be easily removed (using a quick release method) above the venipuncture site. The purpose of the tourniquet is to slow down venous flow away from the puncture site and to not inhibit arterial flow to the puncture site. This causes the vein to enlarge, making it easier to locate and puncture. A tourniquet should not be left on longer than 1 minute because this may change the composition of the blood and make testing inaccurate.

Blood Collection Additives and Collection Tubes

BLOOD COLLECTION ADDITIVES

Anticoagulant and antiglycolytic additives:

Anticoagulant	Antiglycolytic Agent
EDTA	Sodium fluoride
Citrates	Lithium iodoacetate
Heparin	Potassium oxalate
Oxalates	

Additives found with colored tube stoppers:

Yellow	ACD (acid-citrate-dextrose)
Red (glass tube)	None
Light blue	Sodium citrate
Lavender	EDTA
Dark green	Heparin
Gray	Potassium oxalate and sodium fluoride
Gold	Silica, thixotropic gel
Mottled red and gray	Silica, thixotropic gel

EDTA

Ethylenediaminetetraacetic acid (EDTA) is a potassium-based or sodium-based anticoagulant used in blood collection tubes (usually lavender and pink) to prevent clotting of the whole blood specimens (complete blood count [CBC] and blood component tests) and to save specimens for blood bank testing. EDTA binds calcium to prevent clotting, preserves cell morphology, and prevents the aggregation of platelets. The tube should be filled to the specified level, and the correct tube size should be selected for the necessary volume. Immediately after sample collection, 8–10 inversions are needed in order to thoroughly mix EDTA with the blood. Failure to adequately mix them can result in formation of microclots or aggregated platelets. EDTA may be in liquid form (K3EDTA) or spray-dried (K2EDTA), but the liquid form may dilute the sample and alter test results (1–2% decrease). The EDTA tube with the blood sample should be placed in a refrigerator while awaiting processing. The timing and storage requirements vary according to the type of test. For example, red blood cell count remains stable for up to 72 hours under refrigeration, but white blood cell counts are less stable.

HEPARIN

The purpose of heparin is to prevent coagulation. The three types of heparin are ammonium, sodium, and lithium. Ammonium heparin is used for hematocrit determinations and is found in capillary tubes. Sodium heparin and lithium heparin are used in evacuated tubes. Be sure that the heparin being used is not what is being tested. For example, heparin is used for electrolyte testing, but sodium is a commonly tested electrolyte, so sodium heparin would not be an appropriate heparin to use to test for electrolytes. It is important to mix heparin tubes properly to prevent microclots.

> **Review Video: Heparin – An Injectable Anti-Coagulant**
> Visit mometrix.com/academy and enter code: 127426

PPT, SST, AND PST

All three tubes contain thixotropic gel, which is a nonreactive synthetic substance that serves as an actual physical barrier between the serum and the cellular portion of a specimen after the specimen has been centrifuged. If thixotropic gel is used in a tube with EDTA, it is referred to as **a plasma preparation tube (PPT)**. When thixotropic gel is used in the serum collection tube, the gel is referred to as a serum separator, thus the tube and the gel are called the **serum separator tube (SST)**. When thixotropic gel is used in a tube with heparin, it is called a plasma separator. Thus, when thixotropic gel and heparin are in a tube, the tube is called the **plasma separator tube (PST)**.

COLLECTION TUBES BASED ON TEST

BLACK, DARK BLUE, AND LIGHT BLUE

Collection tube	Black	Blue (dark)	Blue (light)
Tests	Erythrocyte sedimentation rate (ESR)	Toxicology, trace metals, nutritional analysis	Coagulation
Additives	Sodium citrate	EDTA, heparin, or none	Sodium citrate
Specimen	Whole blood	Plasma or serum	Plasma
Inversions	0	Heparin or EDTA, 8–10. No additive, 0.	3–4
Department	Hematology	Hematology	Hematology
Notes	Do not invert. Fill tube completely.	Verify additive before proceeding.	Fill tube completely.

GOLD/TIGER-TOP/RED-GRAY, GRAY OR LIGHT GRAY, DARK GREEN

Collection tube	Gold, tiger-top, red-gray	Gray, light gray	Green (dark)
Tests	Blood chemistries, serology, immunology	Lactic acid, glucose tolerance test (GTT), fasting blood sugar (FBS), blood alcohol	Blood chemistry, ammonia, electrolytes, arterial blood gas (ABG)
Additives	Clot activator and/or thixotropic gel	Iodoacetate, sodium fluoride, and/or potassium oxalate or heparin or EDTA	Heparin (sodium)
Specimen	Serum	Plasma	Plasma or whole blood
Inversions	5–6	8–10	8–10
Department	Chemistry	Chemistry	Chemistry
Notes	Also called a serum separator tube	May need to be placed on ice.	STAT test

LIGHT GREEN OR GRAY/GREEN, LAVENDER, AND ORANGE OR YELLOW-GRAY

Collection tube	Light green, gray/green	Lavender	Orange, yellow-gray
Tests	Potassium, chemistry tests	CBC, molecular tests	Chemistry tests
Additives	Heparin (lithium), thixotropic gel	EDTA	Thrombin
Specimen	Plasma	Whole blood	Serum
Inversions	8–10	8–10	8–10
Department	Chemistry	Hematology	Chemistry
Notes		Most common test	STAT test

PINK, RED (GLASS), RED (PLASTIC)

Collection tube	Pink	Red (glass)	Red (plastic)
Tests	Hematology, typing and screening	Chemistry, serology, immunology, crossmatch (for blood bank)	Chemistry, serology
Additives	EDTA	None	Clot activators
Specimen	Whole blood	Serum	Serum
Inversions	8–10	0	0
Department	Blood bank	Chemistry	Chemistry
Notes	Do not confuse pink and lavender tubes.	Specimen must rest 30 minutes. Do not confuse with plastic red tube.	Specimen must rest 30 minutes. Do not confuse with glass red tube.

TAN, STERILE YELLOW, NONSTERILE YELLOW

Collection tube	Tan	Yellow (sterile)	Yellow (nonsterile)
Tests	Lead analysis	Blood culture	Human leukocyte antigen (HLA), paternity test, tissue typing
Additives	K2EDTA	Sodium polyanethol sulfonate (SPS)	Acid-citrate-dextrose (ACD)
Specimen	Plasma	Whole blood	Whole blood
Inversions	8–10	8–10	8–10
Department	Chemistry	Microbiology	Chemistry
Notes		Do not confuse with nonsterile yellow tube.	Do not confuse with sterile yellow tube.

Blood Sample Collection Procedures

PRIORITIZATION OF SPECIMEN COLLECTION AND RESULTS

The nomenclature and scheme for prioritizing specimen collection and results are as follows:

Priority	Discussion
1. STAT, medical emergency, immediate	Patient is in critical condition, or results are needed immediately. Tests include glucose, cardiac enzymes, hemoglobin and hematocrit, and electrolytes. Collect sample immediately and alert laboratory technicians. STAT orders from ED usually have priority over inpatient STAT orders.
2. Timed specimen	Must be obtained as close to the specified time as possible to ensure meaningful results. Tests include 2-hour PP GTT, cortisol, blood cultures, and cardiac enzymes. Note exact time of collection on sample.
3. ASAP (as soon as possible), preop, and postop	Patient is in serious but not critical condition. Tests include hemoglobin and hematocrit, electrolytes, and glucose. Preop is collected before surgery to verify suitability (CBC, platelet function, hemoglobin, hematocrit, partial thromboplastin time [PTT], and type and crossmatch), and postop is collected to assess condition (hemoglobin, hematocrit). Some patients (preop) may be NPO (that is, not allowed to eat or drink anything).
4. Fasting	Verify fasting before collection. Tests include glucose, cholesterol, and triglycerides.
5. Routine	Collect when possible, but there is no urgency to do so because these tests are used to monitor condition or establish diagnosis. Tests include CBC and chemistry panels.

PROPER ANTISEPTIC AGENTS

Antiseptics inhibit organisms but do not kill all of them; however, the disinfectants that are better able to kill organisms are unsafe to use on skin. New recommendations from the Clinical and Laboratory Standards Institute (CLSI) stress the importance of cleaning the venipuncture site with friction as a means to destroy the most bacteria possible (rather than the classic concentric circle method previously recommended). A number of different antiseptics can be used for skin preparation for common phlebotomy tests:

- **Isopropyl alcohol 70%**: This is the most commonly used and recommended antiseptic, as it is tolerated by most individuals and has good antiseptic qualities. It is usually supplied in individually wrapped pads.
- **Ethyl alcohol**: Generally, it needs to be a higher concentration and left on for a longer period of time than isopropyl alcohol.
- **Povidone iodine/tincture of iodine**: Used when higher-order antisepsis is needed, such as for blood cultures. However, many patients are allergic to iodine, so this limits use.
- **Benzalkonium chloride**: May be used as a substitute for alcohol, as indicated for when measuring blood alcohol levels.
- **Chlorhexidine gluconate**: Used when higher-order antisepsis is needed, such as for blood cultures, and recommended for IV catheter sites. Must air-dry completely to be fully effective.

VENIPUNCTURE PROCEDURES

LOCATING VEINS THAT ARE DIFFICULT TO VISUALIZE OR FEEL

When veins are difficult to visualize or feel, different techniques may be used:

- **Massage**: Gently massaging the arm, starting at the wrist and moving proximally to the venipuncture site after applying the tourniquet, may help veins stand out; however, excessive massaging may alter results.
- **Heat application**: Applying a heating pad or a warm moist compress to the site for 5 minutes may help to distend the vein by causing vasodilation, making the vein easier to locate.
- **Fist pumping**: After the tourniquet is applied, the patient should be asked to make a fist, as this helps the veins to appear more prominent. However, repeatedly pumping the fist should be avoided because this may alter some test results (potassium, phosphate), and the movement may make the vein harder to locate.
- **Positioning**: Lowering the arm to a dependent position (such as over the side of the bed) may help to fill the veins and make them easier to locate. Rotating the arm may help to locate a vein.

> **Review Video: <u>Starting and IV</u>**
> Visit mometrix.com/academy and enter code: 380529

APPROPRIATE SITE FOR VENIPUNCTURE

The vein that is most commonly used for **venipuncture** is the median cubital, which joins the cephalic and basilic veins and is easily accessed in the antecubital space of the arm. Other veins that are sometimes used include the cephalic vein and the basilic vein. The basilic vein lies close to the median nerve and should, therefore, be the last choice. Additionally, the proximal portion of the vein lies near arteries, which can result in accidental arterial blood draw and excessive bleeding. The dorsal metacarpal veins in the hands are easily visible and accessible, but should usually be avoided in older adults because of little supporting subcutaneous tissue.

The nerve most often injured with venipuncture is the median nerve because blood draws are most frequently done in the antecubital space, and the median nerve, which is the largest in the arm, passes through this area. The second most common injury is of the radial nerve, which runs near the cephalic vein on the radial side of the wrist and into the palm of the hand.

A last-resort vein would be the basilic vein because it rolls easily and is positioned so that the brachial artery and a major nerve are at risk for puncture if used. Ankle and foot veins should only be punctured at the discretion of a physician and should only be used when no other veins are appropriate. Poor circulation and clotting factors may affect results of tests and cause puncture wounds that may not readily heal. Venipuncture should be avoided in the 7.5 cm area above the thumb and on the palmar surface of the wrist.

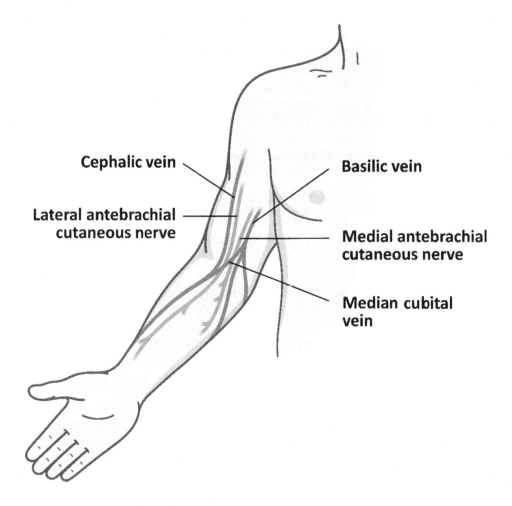

VARIABLES THAT INFLUENCE SITE SELECTION

The following are some variables that make a site **inappropriate** for selection:

1. Injuries to the skin such as burns, scars, and tattoos
2. Damaged veins from repeated collections or drug use
3. Swelling (edema)
4. Hematoma (bruising)
5. Mastectomy or cancer removal, including skin cancer

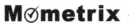

SELECTING EQUIPMENT AFTER IDENTIFYING COLLECTION SITE

Selecting equipment after identifying the collection site allows the clinician to waste less equipment, because if equipment is selected first, the collection site could turn out to be inappropriate for the equipment assembled. Also, this allows for adequate drying time for the alcohol (which is required for proper cleaning of the site and also reduces the sting from the alcohol). A site should have a minimum drying time of 30 seconds.

PERFORMING THE VENIPUNCTURE

After identifying the site, performing appropriate antisepsis, and gathering supplies, the next step in blood collection is anchoring the vein. **Anchoring a vein** involves stretching the skin one inch below the site to provide a taut surface and securing the vein to minimize moving and rolling during puncture. When the puncture site is the antecubital area, the thumb should be placed one to two inches below the antecubital area, pulling the tissue distally with the other fingers wrapped about the back of the arm to secure the arm. It's important to avoid a C-hold—with the thumb below and index finger above the puncture site—because this poses a risk of accidental needlestick if the patient jerks the arm way. If veins on the back of the hand are used, then the patient's hand should be grasped right below the knuckles, the patient's fingers bent, and the skin on the top of the hand stretched taut with the thumb. Most needles are inserted bevel up at an angle of 15–30°, depending on the vein depth, in a proximal direction. A slight decrease in resistance (often characterized as a "pop") is felt when the needle enters the vein.

VENIPUNCTURE IN SPECIAL POPULATIONS

PREFERRED METHOD OF RETRIEVING BLOOD FROM CHILD OR INFANT

Skin puncture (a shallow prick that does not enter a vein) is the preferred method for retrieving blood from a **child or infant** because children have smaller quantities of blood than adults. If enough blood is drawn, it can lead to anemia. Also, a child or infant may be hurt if they need to be restrained during a venipuncture. If a child moves around during venipuncture, it may result in an injury to nerves, veins, and arteries.

The first droplet of blood in a skin puncture contains excess tissue fluid, which may affect test results and should therefore be "wasted." Wasting will also allow the alcohol residue on the skin to be wiped away with the first droplet of blood. That alcohol can hemolyze the blood specimen and keep a round droplet of blood from forming. After wasting the first droplet, massaging around the site should generate a second droplet, which should be collected for testing.

SAFEST PLACE FOR HEEL PUNCTURE IN INFANTS

The National Committee for Clinical Laboratory Standards (NCCLS) states that the safest area for skin puncture in an infant is on the plantar surface of the heel, medial to the imaginary line extending from the middle of the big toe to the heel, or lateral to an imaginary line extending from between the fourth and fifth toes to the heel.

Deep punctures of an infant's heel can lead to osteochondritis (inflammation of the bone and cartilage) and osteomyelitis (inflammation of the bone). Lancets that control the depth of the heel stick should be used when available to avoid this complication.

VENIPUNCTURE ON DIALYSIS PATIENTS

Dialysis patients often have an arteriovenous (AV) shunt or fistula (usually in the forearm) created for dialysis access to filter toxins from the blood. Neither the AV shunt nor the fistula should be used to draw blood, and any blood draw should be on the opposite side. Venipuncture should be minimized in order to save veins, as shunts and fistulas usually have to be periodically replaced. So if patients have advanced kidney disease and may be candidates for dialysis, or already have a shunt or fistula in place, then the dorsal veins of the hands should be used for blood draws, and the cephalic and antecubital veins should be avoided. Draw blood from foot veins only if no other access is available because of increased risk of complications. When possible, capillary blood should be used. If post-dialysis blood values for blood urea nitrogen (BUN), sodium, and calcium are ordered, blood should be drawn within 20 seconds to 2 minutes after discontinuation of dialysis to obtain accurate results. Plasma levels of BUN increase up to 20% within 30 minutes, so timing of the blood draw is critical.

ARTERIAL PUNCTURES
COMMON SITES FOR ARTERIAL PUNCTURE

The **radial artery is the preferred choice for arterial puncture**. It is located on the thumb side of the wrist and is most commonly used. The brachial artery is the second choice. It is located in the medial anterior aspect of the antecubital area near the biceps tendon insertion. The femoral artery is only used by physicians and trained ER personnel. It is usually used in emergency situations or with patients with low cardiac output.

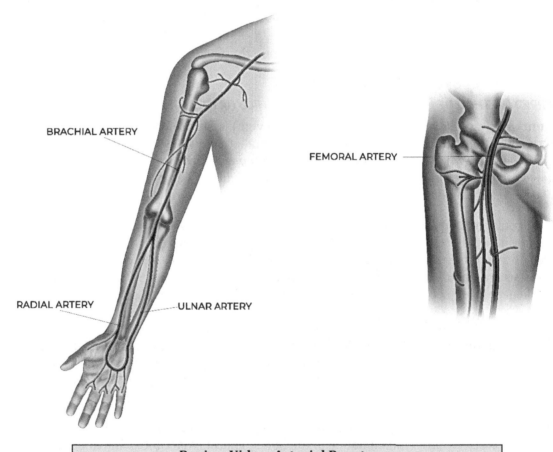

Review Video: Arterial Punctures
Visit mometrix.com/academy and enter code: 112543

ULNAR ARTERY AND THE ALLEN TEST

The purpose of the **Allen test** is to determine the presence of collateral circulation in the hand by the ulnar artery prior to an arterial puncture of the radial artery. The ulnar artery provides collateral circulation for the hand. Since the radial artery is most commonly used in arterial puncture, the ulnar artery is there as a backup to provide blood to the hand if the radial artery is damaged and becomes unable to supply blood to the hand. Ensuring the integrity of the ulnar artery is critical because if the radial artery is damaged and the ulnar artery is not providing sufficient blood flow, there is risk of serious damage to the hand.

The **Allen test** is as follows:

1. Compress the radial and ulnar arteries with the fingers while the patient makes a fist.
2. The patient opens their hand; it should have a blanched appearance.
3. The ulnar artery is released, and the patient's hand should flush with color. If this occurs, the patient has a positive Allen test and has collateral circulation of the ulnar artery.

INVERSION

Inversion (the act of turning a collection tube upside-down and back) is carried out immediately after the blood sample is collected to mix an additive with the blood sample. Tubes without additives do not require inversions. Inversions must be done gently to thoroughly mix the additive with the sample. It's important to avoid shaking the tube or inverting too vigorously because this may result in hemolysis of the sample. If hemolysis occurs, then a number of different tests cannot be performed on the sample, including electrolyte and enzyme tests. If the inversions are done inadequately and the additive is not thoroughly mixed with the sample, microclots may develop, which could interfere with hematology tests. If inversion of gel separation tubes does not result in thorough mixing, this may interfere with clotting. The number of inversions needed varies according to the type of test and the type of additive, but most additives require 8–10 inversions.

PREFERRED ORDER OF DRAW

Blood collection tubes must be drawn in a specific order to avoid cross-contamination of additives between tubes. The **recommended order** of draw is:

1. **Blood culture tube** (yellow-black stopper).
2. **Coagulation tube** (light blue stopper, sodium citrate additive). If a routine coagulation assay is the only test ordered, then a single light blue stopper tube may be drawn. If there is a concern regarding contamination by tissue fluids or thromboplastins, then you may draw a non-additive tube first, and then the light blue stopper. This sample must be filled completely to the fill line in order to be analyzed.
3. **Non-additive tube** (red stopper or SST).
4. **Additive tubes** in this order:
   a. Serum separator tube (SST, red-gray or gold stopper). Contains a gel separator and clot activator.
   b. Sodium heparin (dark green stopper).
   c. Plasma separator tube (PST, light green stopper). Contains lithium heparin anticoagulant and a gel separator.
   d. EDTA (lavender stopper).
   e. ACDA or ACDB (pale yellow stopper). Contains acid-citrate-dextrose.
   f. Oxalate/fluoride (light gray stopper).

Post Care of Venous, Arterial, and Capillary Puncture Sites

Post care for blood collection sites includes:

- **Venous**: Place a folded gauze square over the puncture site, apply manual pressure for 1–2 minutes until bleeding stops (longer if necessary), and then cover with a pressure dressing or adhesive bandage.
- **Arterial**: Place a folded gauze square over the puncture site and apply manual pressure for 3–5 minutes (longer with anticoagulation or coagulopathy). If bleeding, swelling, or bruising persists after the initial period of manual pressure, continue pressure for an additional 2 minutes before checking again. The pressure should be maintained until all bleeding has stopped. A pressure bandage should never be used in lieu of manual pressure, and the patient should not apply pressure. Once bleeding stops, clean the area with povidone iodine or chlorhexidine and check again in two minutes. Check distal pulse. If unable to find a pulse after an arterial puncture or if the pulse is faint, blood flow may be blocked partially or completely by a blood clot. Notify the patient's nurse or physician STAT so that circulation can begin to be restored as quickly as possible. Finally, apply pressure dressing.
- **Capillary**: Apply pressure with a clean piece of gauze over the puncture site until bleeding stops. Because the puncture is so small, a bandage is not usually required but can be applied.

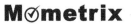

Specific Blood Tests

BLOOD CULTURES

Blood collection for blood cultures usually involves collecting samples in two containers:

- **Aerobic container**: Contains air and a medium to encourage growth of aerobic organisms.
- **Anaerobic container**: A vacuum that contains no air but contains a medium to encourage growth of anaerobic organisms.

Blood cultures may be used to determine the cause of fever of unknown origin and to determine if bacteremia is present. If a needle and syringe are used to collect the specimen, the anaerobic container is filled first, and then the aerobic container. If a winged infusion set ("butterfly") is used, then the aerobic bottle is filled first because the tubing may contain a small amount of air. If multiple sets are ordered at the same time, each set must be obtained either from a separate site, or by waiting 30 minutes between obtaining specimens (with fresh punctures for each collection). Blood culture specimens cannot be taken from preexisting peripheral or central intravenous catheters unless they are taken immediately upon the insertion of the IV.

BLOOD CULTURE PROCESS

The general blood culture collection process is as follows:

1. Verify patient identification with two identifiers.
2. Use standard precautions and venipuncture procedures, and use aseptic technique when handling equipment to avoid contamination.
3. Vigorously scrub skin with antiseptic (chlorhexidine gluconate, or CHG, is most widely recommended) for 30–60 seconds to remove skin bacteria, and allow to dry.
4. Swab caps of blood culture bottles with antiseptic. Note fill line.
5. Carry out blood draw. Adults: 10–20 mL per set, Pediatric patients: 1–2 mL per set.
6. If multiple draws are ordered, wait 30 minutes between draws unless otherwise ordered. Take multiple draws from different sites if possible.
7. Replace venipuncture needle with blunt fill needle and use transfer device.
8. Inject blood culture specimen into both anaerobic and aerobic bottles.
9. Mix specimen with medium in the culture bottle according to directions.
10. Label culture bottles.
11. Dispose of contaminated equipment and sharps in appropriate containers.
12. Remove gloves, sanitize hands, and transport specimen to the laboratory. Incubate and monitor per protocol.

TYPE AND ANTIBODY SCREEN OR CROSSMATCH

Type and antibody screen or crossmatch to determine blood type and compatibility may be performed for many reasons, while crossmatches are usually performed only for elective surgeries during which blood loss is probable. Type and screen (indirect Coombs test) identifies the blood type by identifying the A, B, and Rh antigens and by screening for particular antibodies most commonly implicated in non-ABO hemolytic reactions. Type and screen is more often performed for procedures that result in <10% transfusions. Crossmatching (mixing donor and recipient blood to observe for agglutination) includes testing for immunoglobulin G antibodies and is performed if blood loss is probable. In emergencies, type-specific and partially crossmatched blood may be used, because this procedure takes less than 5 minutes. Otherwise, type-specific non-crossmatched blood is used, and as a last resort, type O-negative packed red blood cells are administered.

ETHANOL (BLOOD ALCOHOL) TEST

Ethanol (EtOH) tests, commonly referred to as blood alcohol tests, may be done for clinical or legal reasons. If carried out for legal reasons, such as to determine whether a driver was under the influence of alcohol, chain-of-custody protocols must be followed and carefully documented. Special considerations include the following:

- Skin antiseptics containing alcohol (isopropyl alcohol, methanol, tincture of iodine) cannot be used because they may contaminate the specimen and alter test results. Alternative skin antiseptics include povidone iodine and aqueous benzalkonium chloride. If no alternative is available, the site should be thoroughly washed with soap and water and dried.
- Alcohol readily evaporates, so the collection tube should be completely filled and the stopper should be left on the tube until ready to perform testing.
- Testing may be done on whole blood, serum, or plasma. A glass gray-top sodium fluoride tube, with or without anticoagulant, is usually used.

RED BLOOD CELLS

Red blood cells (RBCs or erythrocytes) are biconcave disks that contain **hemoglobin** (95% of mass), which carries oxygen throughout the body. The heme portion of the cell contains **iron**, which binds to the oxygen. RBCs live about 120 days, after which they are destroyed and their hemoglobin is recycled or excreted.

The **morphology** of RBCs may vary depending on the type of anemia:

- Size: Normocytes, microcytes, macrocytes.
- Shape: Spherocytes (round), poikilocytes (irregular), drepanocytes (sickled).
- Color (reflecting concentration of hemoglobin): Normochromic, hypochromic.

Hemoglobin measures the amount of oxygen-carrying hemoglobin protein in the blood, and **hematocrit** measures the percentage of RBCs in whole blood.

Collection and purpose are the same: Whole blood is collected in a lavender-topped EDTA tube, in a microtainer (capillary tube), or in a green-topped lithium or sodium-heparin tube. The sample should be inverted 6–8 times immediately after a blood draw. This test is done to assess anemia, hydration, polycythemia, and blood loss, and to monitor therapy.

Normal hemoglobin values

- Adult male: 13.2–17.3 g/dL
- Adult female: 11.7–15.5 g/dL
- Critical values: <6.6 or >20 g/dL

Normal hematocrit values

- Adult male: 38–51%
- Adult female: 33–45%
- Critical values (adults): <19.8% or >60%

Reticulocyte count: Measures marrow production and should rise with anemia. Normal values: 0.5–1.5% of total RBCs.

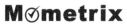

WBC Count and Differential

White blood cell (leukocyte) count is used as an indicator of bacterial and viral infection. **WBC count** is reported as the total number of all white blood cells.

- Normal WBC for adults: 4,800–10,000
- Acute infection: 10,000+
- Severe infection: 30,000
- Viral infection: 4,000 and below

The **differential** provides the percentage of each different type of leukocyte. An increase in the white blood cell count is usually related to an increase in one type. Often, an increase in immature neutrophils (bands), referred to as a "shift to the left," is an indication of an infectious process:

- Normal immature neutrophils (bands): 1–3%. Increase with infection.
- Normal segmented neutrophils (segs) for adults: 50–62%. Increase with acute, localized, or systemic bacterial infections.
- Normal eosinophils: 0–3%. Decrease with stress and acute infection.
- Normal basophils: 0–1%. Decrease during acute stage of infection.
- Normal lymphocytes: 25–40%. Increase in some viral and bacterial infections.
- Normal monocytes: 3–7%. Increase during recovery stage of acute infection.

Normal Arterial Blood pH

pH is the measure of the acidity of a solution. pH is equal to the negative logarithm of the concentration of hydrogen ions in a solution. Generally speaking, a pH of 7 is neutral. Values less than 7 are considered acidic, and values greater than 7 are considered basic. A range of 6.5–7.5 is considered a neutral environment.

The normal range for **arterial blood pH** is 7.35–7.45. Acidosis is characterized by below-normal blood pH. Alkalosis is characterized by above-normal blood pH. This blood sample must be taken from an artery, as venous pH is not as accurate in assessing an individual's pH balance (although it is a secondary option if an arterial sample is not possible). Arterial samples can be collected using a straight stick, or by drawing off of an arterial line if the patient has this access.

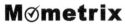

ENDOCRINE SYSTEM BLOOD TESTS

Endocrine system blood tests include:

- **Aldosterone**: Aldosterone is a mineralocorticoid produced by adrenal glands in response to increased potassium, decreased sodium, or decreased blood volume. It helps to regulate sodium and potassium levels. The specimen is collected with a plain red-top tube and tested on serum (refrigerate after centrifugation). This is an "upright" sample, meaning it should be obtained after patient has been in a sitting (upright) position for at least 30 minutes.
- **Renin**: Renin is an enzymatic hormone secreted by the kidneys in response to sodium depletion. It is tested to determine the cause of hypertension. This test is usually conducted along with aldosterone level. The specimen is collected in a lavender-topped EDTA or pink-topped EDTA tube and is conducted on plasma.
- **Cortisol**: This is the primary glucocorticoid secreted by adrenal glands. It stimulates gluconeogenesis, serves as an insulin antagonist, suppresses inflammatory response, and mobilizes proteins and fats. This test assesses adrenal function and is used to diagnose Cushing's disease and Addison's disease. Specimen collected for the serum test is in the red- or red/gray-topped tube, and specimen for plasma tests is in the green-topped heparin tube. If serial tests are required, the same type of tube should be used for all tests. Time of draw must be correctly noted. Tests are often done at 8 AM and 4 PM.
- **Glucagon**: This hormone is produced in the pancreas and excreted by kidneys, increasing the amount of glucose and fat in the blood. Specimen collected is in a chilled lavender-topped EDTA tube, and the test is conducted on plasma. Specimen must be tightly capped and placed in ice slurry for transport.
- **Insulin**: This hormone is produced in the beta cells of the pancreas. It regulates metabolism of proteins, fats, and carbohydrates, and controls production and storage of glucose. This test is done to determine the amount of insulin secreted in response to glucose and may include the administration of a standardized dose of glucose at fixed time periods. The specimen is collected in a red-topped tube, and the test is conducted on serum.
- **Erythropoietin** (EPO): This hormone is produced in the kidney and promotes red cell production. The test assesses the cause of anemia and/or kidney function. The specimen is collected in a red-, gold-, or red/gray-top tube, and the test is conducted on serum. Phlebotomy may increase levels of EPO.

COAGULATION TESTS AND PROCEDURE

Test [normal range]	Procedure
Fibrinogen (factor I) [100–400 mg/dL]	Collect 1 mL blood in sodium citrate blue-capped tube (completely filled) for photo-optical clot detection. Synthesized in the liver, it converts to fibrin, which combines with platelets in coagulation sequence. **Increased:** Acute myocardial infarction (MI), cancer, eclampsia, multiple myeloma, Hodgkin's disease, nephrotic syndrome, tissue trauma. **Decreased:** Disseminated intravascular coagulation (DIC), liver disease, congenital fibrinogen abnormality.
Fibrin degradation product (fibrin split products or FSPs) [<5 mcg/mL FEU*]	Collect 1 mL blood in sodium citrate blue-capped tube (completely filled) for latex agglutination test. Transport frozen. FSPs occur as clots form and more breakdown of fibrinogen and fibrin occurs, interfering with blood coagulation by coating platelets and disrupting thrombin, and attaching to fibrinogen so stable clots can't form. **Increased:** DIC, liver disease, MI, hemorrhage, pulmonary embolism, renal disease, obstetric complications, kidney transplant rejection.
Heparin assay (antithrombin III) [1–3 mo: 48–108% 1–5 yr: 82–139% 6–17 yr: 90–131% >18 yr: 80–120%]	Collect 1 mL blood in sodium citrate blue-capped tube (completely filled) for chromogenic immunoturbidimetry. Used to diagnose heparin resistance in patients receiving heparin therapy and to diagnose hypercoagulable conditions. **Increased:** Acute hepatitis, kidney transplantation, vitamin K deficiency. **Decreased:** DIC, liver transplantation, nephrotic syndrome, pulmonary embolism, venous thrombosis, liver failure, cirrhosis, carcinoma.
Platelet aggregation [results vary]	Collect 4–5 mL sample in sodium citrate tubes for analysis with light transmission aggregometer. Must be processed within 60 minutes of collection. Test measures the ability of platelets to aggregate and form clots in response to various activators. **Decreased:** Myeloproliferative disorders, autoimmune disorders, uremia, clotting disorders, and adverse effects of medications. Drugs that affect clotting should be avoided before a test for up to two weeks (on advice of physician).
Prothrombin time (PT) [10–14 seconds]	Collect 1 mL blood in sodium citrate blue-capped tube (completely filled). **Increased:** Anticoagulation therapy, vitamin K deficiency, decreased prothrombin, DIC, liver disease, and malignant neoplasm. Some drugs may shorten time. **Critical value:** >27 seconds.
Partial thromboplastin time (PTT) [60–70 seconds]	Collect 1 mL blood in sodium citrate blue-capped tube (completely filled). **Increased:** Hemophilia A & B, von Willebrand's, vitamin deficiency, lupus, DIC, and liver disease. **Critical value:** >100 seconds.
Activated partial thromboplastin time (aPTT) [30–40 seconds]	Collect 1 mL blood in sodium citrate blue-capped tube (completely filled). Similar to PTT, but an activator is added that speeds clotting time. Used to monitor heparin dosage. **Increased:** Same as for PTT. **Decreased:** Extensive cancer, early DIC, and after acute hemorrhage. **Critical value:** >70 seconds.
D-dimer [0.5 mcg/mL (measuring fibrinogen equivalent units)]	Collect 1 mL blood in sodium citrate blue-capped tube (completely filled) for immunoturbidimetry. Transport frozen. D-dimer is a specific polymer that results when fibrin breaks down, giving a marker to indicate the degree of fibrinolysis. **Increased:** DIC, pulmonary embolism, deep vein thrombosis, late pregnancy, neoplastic disorder, preeclampsia, arterial/venous thrombosis.

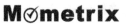

C-Reactive Protein and Erythrocyte Sedimentation Rate

C-reactive protein is an acute-phase reactant produced by the liver in response to inflammation that causes neutrophils, granulocytes, and macrophages to secrete cytokines. Thus, levels of **C-reactive protein** rise when there is inflammation or infection. It has been found to be a helpful measure of response to treatment for pyoderma gangrenosum ulcers:

- Normal values: 2.6–7.6 μg/dL

Erythrocyte sedimentation rate (sed rate) measures the distance erythrocytes fall in a vertical tube of anticoagulated blood in one hour. Because fibrinogen—which increases in response to infection—also increases the rate of the fall, the sed rate can be used as a nonspecific test for inflammation when infection is suspected. The sed rate is sensitive to osteomyelitis and may be used to monitor treatment response. Values vary according to gender and age:

- <50: Males 0–15 mm/hr. Females 0–20 mm/hr
- >50: Males 0–20 mm/hr. Females 0–30 mm/hr

Trace and Ultratrace Elements

Trace elements are metals and may include iron, lead, zinc, mercury, aluminum, and copper. Ultratrace elements include boron, nickel, vanadium, arsenic, and silicon. Specimens may easily be contaminated, so care must be taken to avoid any specimen containers with metal. Special trace-element-free specimen tubes (usually royal blue and containing EDTA, heparin, or no additive) should be used because trace metals may be found in standard glass and plastic tubes and in the stoppers. Because some substances—gadolinium, iodine, and barium contrast—interfere with test results, testing should be delayed for at least 96 hours if patients have received any of these. The specimens must be kept clean and protected from dust. No iodine products should be used for antisepsis, only alcohol. When transferring plasma or serum, it must be poured into aliquots and not transferred by a pipette. Labels are color-coded to indicate the type of additive: lavender indicates EDTA, green indicates heparin, and red indicates no additive.

BASAL STATE REQUIREMENTS FOR BLOOD TESTS

Some tests need to be carried out during a patient's **basal state**, which is the state the body is in when the patient awakes in the morning after 12 hours of fasting (no nutritional intake, although water is usually allowed). In practice, patients are usually asked to fast for 8 to 12 hours, depending on the test. In addition to fasting, patients should be advised to avoid smoking, chewing any kind of gum, or exercising, as these may alter the patient's basal state and affect test results. In some cases, patients may be asked to abstain from alcohol or drugs for a period of time (often the day before the test). Tests that are usually done after fasting include:

- Glucose: 8 hours
- Triglycerides: 9–12 hours
- Lipids: 9–12 hours
- Renal function tests: 8–12 hours
- Vitamin B12 test: 6–8 hours
- Basic/comprehensive metabolic panels: 10–12 hours
- Gamma-glutamyl transferase test: 8 hours
- Iron levels: 12 hours

FACTORS INFLUENCING BASAL STATE

Factors that influence the basal state include the following:

- Age
- Altitude
- Daily variations
- Dehydration
- Diet
- Drugs (prescription and illegal)
- Exercise
- Fever
- Gender
- Humidity
- Jaundice
- Position
- Pregnancy
- Smoking
- Stress
- Temperature

Point of Care Tests

WAIVED TESTING

While laboratory testing is regulated by the Clinical Laboratory Improvement Amendments (CLIA) and results are monitored through proficiency testing, some tests are considered to have a very low risk of error (although they are not necessarily error free), and the patient is unlikely to experience harm if a result is in error. These tests do not require proficiency testing. **Waived testing** includes specific tests exempted by CLIA regulations, tests approved by the FDA for home use (such as pregnancy tests), and tests for which the FDA has applied a waiver based on CLIA regulations and guidelines. Labs that carry out only waived testing must obtain a CLIA Certificate of Waiver (COW). Waived tests include dipstick or tablet reagent tests (such as for bilirubin and ketones), fecal-occult blood tests, blood glucose monitoring strips, ovulation tests (color-based), ESR tests, blood counts, and hemoglobin. Some states may require proficiency testing for tests that are waived under CLIA regulations, and some laboratories may choose to have proficiency testing of waived tests for internal quality control.

SPECIFIC POINT-OF-CARE TESTS

Point-of-care tests may give qualitative results (present or absent, such as a pregnancy test) or quantitative results (precise numbers, such as glucose). Quality control is critical in ensuring that test results are accurate, and those performing the tests must be well-trained. Advantages include rapid turnaround time and small sample volumes. Additionally, a sample does not require pre-processing. Disadvantages include increased cost, quality variation, and billing concerns. Tests include:

- **Glucose**: A glucometer is used with a drop of blood from a finger. The drop is obtained with a lancet, applied to a strip, and inserted into the properly calibrated glucometer, which reports the results. Normal values for a child range from 60 to 100 mg/dL, and for an adult, under 100 mg/dL (fasting usually ranges from 70 to 100 mg/dL). Critical values are less than 40 g/dL or greater than 400 mg/dL. Non-glucose sugars, such as those in peritoneal dialysate, can affect results.
- **Coagulation**: Point-of-care tests for coagulation use a sample of whole blood to provide the patient's PT, aPTT, and international normalized ratio (INR) for patients on warfarin anticoagulant. Some devices can measure activated clotting time (ACT) for patients on unfractionated heparin. For example, the CoaguChek XS is a handheld meter used to monitor INR. A sample of capillary blood is obtained, and a drop of blood is placed on a test strip. The test strip must be inserted into the device within 15 seconds. Coagulation measurement begins, and the results are displayed. Test results for these devices are comparable to standard testing.
  - **INR**: (PT result/normal average): <2 for those not receiving anticoagulation and 2–3 for those receiving anticoagulation. Critical value: >3–5 in patients receiving anticoagulation therapy.
- **Pregnancy (human chorionic gonadotropin detection)**: Pregnancy tests are most accurate after a missed period and with the first morning urination. The patient should hold the testing stick in the stream of urine, or dip it in a cup of fresh urine. After the allotted wait time, the testing stick indicates whether the person is pregnant or not. False negatives may occur in early pregnancy.

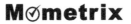

Phlebotomy Complications

ISSUES THAT AFFECT BLOOD COLLECTION

Various issues can affect the blood collection process and lead to complications. Many patients have allergies. These include possible allergies to adhesives, latex, and antiseptics. A patient may have a bleeding or bruising disorder that results from a genetic reason or medication that they are taking. Some patients may faint (syncope) during a procedure. It is very appropriate to recline a patient or have them lie down if they have fainted before. Some patients have a fear of needles. Some may experience nausea and vomiting from fear or an illness they have. It may be necessary to have a trash can or spit-up container nearby for easy access. If a patient is overweight or obese, collection may be difficult.

VASOVAGAL REACTION

A vasovagal reaction, characterized by hypotension, diaphoresis, syncope, and nausea, may occur when a patient receives a venipuncture. If a patient complains of feeling faint and appears suddenly pale and shaky during a venipuncture (a vasovagal reaction characterized by diaphoresis and hypotension), the initial response should be to remove the needle, because if the patient faints and falls, the needle could be dislodged, resulting in trauma. As soon as the needle is removed, sitting patients should be assisted to put their heads low, between their legs. However, the patient is at risk of a fall injury, so the phlebotomist must support the patient. If the patient is in bed, the head of the bed should be lowered. If the patient faints and falls, an incident report must be completed and the patient examined and treated for any injury. The patient may need time to recuperate before another venipuncture is attempted.

NAUSEA AND VOMITING

Patients may experience nausea and vomiting before, during, or after venipuncture because of a nervous response, vasovagal reaction, or current illness. If a patient complains of nausea before the venipuncture begins, the phlebotomist should wait until the symptoms subside unless it is an emergent situation. An emesis basin should be provided for the patient, and the patient should be encouraged to take slow, deep breaths to help relax. In some cases, applying a cold damp cloth to the patient's forehead may help. If the patient begins to vomit during venipuncture, the procedure should be stopped immediately, and a nurse should be called to assist the patient. The patient should be offered tissues to wipe the mouth and water to rinse the mouth (unless NPO). Some tests may induce nausea in patients, such as the glucose tolerance test.

COMPLICATIONS IN PATIENTS WITH CLOTTING DEFICIENCIES

Patients who have clotting deficiencies or who are on anticoagulant therapy, such as warfarin or heparin, may **bleed excessively** after venipuncture. Patients are especially at risk for hematomas and persistent bleeding after venipuncture. Steady and prolonged pressure must be applied until bleeding stops. Elevating the arm may help to slow bleeding. Continue maintaining pressure; only when bleeding has completely stopped may a pressure dressing be applied and left in place for 20–30 minutes, as a precaution. Care must be taken to avoid excessive pressure, which may increase bruising. The phlebotomist should be aware that stroke and heart patients (such as those with atrial fibrillation) often take anticoagulants and should question medications. **Petechiae** may be a sign that a patient has a clotting deficiency, so the phlebotomist should examine the patient's skin carefully and be alert for excessive bleeding after venipuncture.

HEMATOMA

During a venipuncture, if the needle goes through the vein and a **hematoma** begins to rapidly develop, the next step is to remove the needle and tourniquet and apply pressure to prevent further

77

loss of blood into the tissue. A hematoma may also form if the needle only partially penetrates the vessel wall, allowing blood to leak into the tissue. If blood flow stops and a small hematoma begins to form, the needle's bevel may be up against a vessel wall, so rotating it slightly may stop the leak and allow blood to flow into the collection tube. If a very small hematoma is evident during venipuncture, the best initial response is to observe the site and complete the venipuncture. If, however, the hematoma is large or expanding, then the phlebotomist should remove the needle, elevate the arm above the level of the heart, and apply pressure until the bleeding stops. Small hematomas are fairly common, especially in older adults whose veins may be friable and those taking anticoagulants and certain other drugs.

HEMATOMA CAUSES

Hematomas most often result from the following:

- Inadequate pressure to the collection site after a blood draw
- Blood leaking through the back of a vein that was pierced
- Blood leaking from a partially pierced vein
- An artery that was pierced

NERVE INJURY AND SEIZURES

Nerve injury can occur when the needle touches a nerve during a venipuncture, usually the result of poor site selection, improper insertion of needle, or patient movement. The pain is acute, and the patient will generally call out and complain of severe pain, tingling, or "electric shock." The phlebotomist must immediately remove the needle to prevent further damage. Once the bleeding is controlled, an ice pack applied to the site may help to decrease inflammation and pain. The phlebotomist must fill out an incident report and must follow procedures in accordance with facility protocols. Pain may persist for an extended period, and some patients may require physical therapy if nerve damage is severe.

Seizures are an uncommon complication and generally unrelated to venipuncture; however, if a seizure occurs, the phlebotomist should immediately discontinue the venipuncture, apply pressure to the insertion site without restraining the patient, and call for help. The phlebotomist should try to prevent harm to the patient. If the patient is seated, the patient may need to be eased onto the floor with assistance. Place the patient side-lying on their left side if possible.

EDEMA AND PRIOR MASTECTOMY

Blood should not be drawn from edematous tissue because the **edema** may result in the blood being diluted with tissue fluids. Edema is often most pronounced in the hands and feet, but arms may be edematous as well. With generalized edema, the phlebotomist should try to find the least edematous site for venipuncture, should apply gentle pressure to the site to displace the fluid if possible, and should note on the label that edema was present.

Blood generally should not be obtained on the side of a **mastectomy**, regardless of the length of time since surgery, because the circulation may be impaired, and edema may be present. Any degree of lymphedema may alter the results of the blood tests, and the patient is at increased risk of infection from venipuncture. If no other site is available, then a physician's order should be obtained regarding use of this site. With a double mastectomy—especially if any degree of lymphedema is evident—alternative sites, such as feet and legs, may need to be considered. If possible, a sample may be obtained through capillary puncture for lymphedema, but for generalized edema, the sample will be diluted.

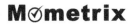

PRE-EXISTING INTRAVENOUS LINE

Blood samples should not be obtained from an **existing intravenous line** because the sample may be contaminated with IV fluids/drugs or diluted. Additionally, the sample is more likely to undergo hemolysis and need to be discarded.

Blood should also not be drawn from the same side as an IV line if possible. If blood must be drawn from an arm that has an intravenous line in place, the IV should be clamped for at least two minutes before the specimen is collected to allow the IV fluid to enter the circulation and reduce the dilution of the blood sample. It is preferable to do the venipuncture at least 5 inches distal to the IV insertion site when possible, with the tourniquet also applied distal to the IV insertion site. The site (proximal or distal) in relation to the IV should be documented.

ALLERGIES

Patients should be questioned about allergies prior to having blood withdrawn. **Common allergies** that may pose a problem include:

- **Latex**: Reactions range from mild to severe anaphylaxis, and latex allergies are increasingly common for those with frequent contact with healthcare, especially those with multiple surgeries and those with spina bifida. The phlebotomist should avoid taking any latex items—such as tourniquets and bandaging supplies—near the patient with a severe allergy, and should generally replace latex items with non-latex for all patients.
- **Iodine**: Patients may be allergic to any skin antiseptic, but allergy to iodine is most common. Patients who report being allergic to fish are also at risk for iodine allergy. Alternative antiseptics should be used in place of antiseptics with iodine.
- **Adhesive**: Some patients are allergic to adhesive, which may cause itching and rash. Some types of tape, such as paper tape, are better tolerated but may still cause a problem for some patients. Stretch bandaging materials (such as Coban) may be used to secure a dressing.

MEDICATIONS AND RECENT SURGERY

Medications that pose a particular concern with phlebotomy are those that interfere with clotting mechanisms:

- **Platelet inhibitors**, such as aspirin and clopidogrel (Plavix)
- **Anticoagulants**, including:
    - Injectable drugs such as heparin, argatroban, and bivalirudin
    - Oral anticoagulants, such as warfarin (Coumadin), rivaroxaban (Xarelto) and dabigatran (Pradaxa)

All of these drugs increase the risk of bleeding, so multiple venipunctures should be avoided when possible. Care must be taken to apply pressure until all bleeding stops, and a compression dressing may then be left in place for at least 20 minutes to ensure no recurrence of bleeding.

Recent surgery may pose a risk of complications, depending on the type of surgery and the medications given to the patient after surgery. Blood should not be drawn from an arm that has recently undergone any type of surgical procedure, or the arm on the side of a mastectomy or any surgery that might interfere with blood flow or lymph flow.

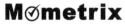

DEHYDRATION AND CHEMOTHERAPY

Dehydration may occur in patients with severe nausea and vomiting and/or diarrhea and those with inadequate fluid intake for body needs. **Dehydration** results in decreased cardiac output and blood volume, so blood vessels constrict, making it difficult to access the veins and resulting in hemoconcentration that affects test results. If possible, the blood draw should be delayed until the patient is more hydrated, but if it is necessary to draw blood, a warm compress may help to dilate the vessels slightly. A smaller-gauge needle or a winged infusion set may also be necessary. The label should indicate that the patient is dehydrated, and the physician should be notified.

Patients on **chemotherapy** often have central lines, such as ports or peripherally inserted central catheter (PICC) lines, and these may, at times, be used to withdraw samples, but phlebotomists are generally prohibited from drawing specimens through central lines. Veins may be fragile and collapse easily, so a smaller-gauge needle or winged infusion set may be necessary. Warming the site may help to make the veins more visible. Edema may obscure veins, and prolonged bleeding may occur because of coagulopathy.

GERIATRICS

Drawing blood from geriatric patients poses a number of challenges:

- **Disabilities**: Patients may be hard of hearing and/or have difficulty speaking, interfering with communication with the patient. The phlebotomist should speak clearly without shouting and allow the patient extra time to respond or indicate comprehension. For patients with vision impairment, the phlebotomist should guide the patient and explain all actions verbally. If a patient has dementia, the phlebotomist should speak in simple sentences and reassure the patient, asking for help if the patient is hostile or combative. Physical disabilities (arthritis, neuromuscular diseases, contractures) may limit mobility.
- **Aging**: Loose skin and loss of muscle tissue may make it difficult to anchor a vein, and veins may be sclerosed or rolling, so careful anchoring of the vein is necessary. Scarred, sclerosed veins should be avoided. Circulation may be impaired (especially with diabetic patients), and medications (such as anticoagulants) may increase bleeding or interfere with test results. Prolonged pressure may need to be applied to puncture sites, and heavy adhesives may tear skin.

OBESITY

Obesity can pose a problem for venipuncture because the patient's veins may be deep and not visible or palpable. The median cubital vein in the antecubital area should be examined first, as it may be palpable between folds of tissue. However, with obese patients, the cephalic vein is often easier to palpate than the median cubital vein. Rotating the hand into prone position (palm down) may make the cephalic vein more palpable. In some cases, a longer needle may be necessary for venipuncture. If there is no or little fat pad on the top of the hand, then the hand veins may be used for venipuncture. Tourniquets may be difficult to position, as they tend to roll and twist. An extra-large tourniquet or Velcro closure strap should be used if possible, but if those are not available, using two tourniquets—one on top of the other—may help keep the tourniquet from twisting. Patients may know from past experience which access site is best, so the phlebotomist should ask the patient directly.

Special Collections

Collection and Preservation of Extravascular Body Fluids for Chemical Analysis

Collection and preservation procedures for the chemical analysis of extravascular body fluids is dependent on fluid type.

Amniotic fluid	The sample is collected by a physician during amniocentesis. Store in a special container (protected from light) at room temperature for chromosome analysis or on ice for some chemistry tests (according to protocol).
Cerebrospinal fluid	The sample is collected by a physician. Collect in 3 tubes (first for culture and others for chemistry and microscopy) and store at room temperature with immediate delivery to lab. *Neisseria meningitidis* is fragile and cold sensitive, so do not chill the specimen.
Gastric fluids	The sample is collected during gastroscopy or from nasogastric (NG) tube. Store in a sterile container at room temperature for up to 6 hours, refrigerated for up to 7 days, and frozen for up to 30 days.
Nasopharyngeal secretions	Collected with swab from nasopharyngeal area. Place swab in tube with transport medium.
Saliva	Collected in a sterile container after the patient rinses their mouth and waits a few minutes. Test immediately (point of care) or freeze for hormone tests to maintain stability.
Semen	Collect a fresh sample from the individual immediately following ejaculation into a sterile container. Keep the sample warm and deliver immediately for testing.
Serous fluid	The sample is collected by a physician, typically through thoracentesis or paracentesis. Samples are labeled as pleural, peritoneal, or pericardial. Place in a sterile container for culture and sensitivity testing (C&S), an EDTA tube for cell counts/smears, and oxalate or fluoride tubes for chemistry tests.
Synovial fluid	The sample is collected by a physician through aspiration of the joint. Place in EDTA or heparin tube for cell counts, smear, and crystal identification; sterile tube for C&S; and plain tube for chemistry and immunology tests.
Sputum	First morning production of sputum preferred because a larger volume is likely to be produced after sleeping. Patients should remove any dentures and rinse mouth before attempting to cough up specimen. Transport at room temperature and process immediately.
Urine	Collected in a sterile container from midstream urination or catheterization. If for 24-hour quantitative testing, urine is collected in a 2L container. Store at room temperature in a sterile container for 2 hours (protected from light) and then refrigerate. If both urinalysis (UA) and C&S are required, then test or refrigerate immediately.

81

Oropharyngeal and Nasopharyngeal Swabs

When obtaining an oropharyngeal or nasopharyngeal swab, the first steps are to wash the hands and don personal protective equipment, including gloves, a mask, and goggles (especially important if the patient is coughing). Seat the patient upright or with the head of the bed elevated to at least 45° and the head tipped back (pillows behind shoulders):

- **Oropharyngeal**: Depress the anterior third of the tongue with the tongue blade and insert the swab without touching the lips, teeth, inside of cheeks, or tongue. Swab both tonsillar areas, moving the swab side to side (including any inflamed areas), and carefully remove the swab, avoiding contact with other tissues. Insert into sterile collection tube, break off stick, secure, and label.
- **Nasopharyngeal**: After the patient blows their nose, ask the patient to occlude one nostril at a time and exhale through the nose to determine if nostrils are clear. Carefully insert the swab through the nose (or nasal speculum if necessary) to the inflamed tissue, rotate the swab in the tissue, and remove the swab without touching other nasal tissue or the speculum. Save as above.

Collection of Stool Specimens

Stool specimens are obtained by placing a stool collection device in a toilet or in a bedpan. The specimen is then placed in a clean specimen container, or if for cultures, in a sterile container. Different types of containers may be used, with or without preservatives, depending on the type of tests being conducted. The sample is transferred using a tongue depressor to the fill-line indicated on the container. If an additive is in the container, the sample should be shaken to mix contents. The container should be properly labeled and sealed in a biohazard bag for transport. For a stool culture, the specimen should be collected before the patient begins antibiotics. The stool specimen is placed in a sterile container, or a cotton-tipped swab is inserted into the rectum and rotated to obtain a fecal sample. Then the swab is inserted into a sterile tube. Stool specimens should be processed as soon as possible or stored at 4° C if there will be a delay of more than two hours before processing.

AFP

AFP is **alpha-fetoprotein**. Normally it is found in the human fetus, but abnormal levels of AFP may indicate a neural tube defect in an infant or other fetal developmental problems. The test is performed on maternal serum. If results are abnormal, a test on the amniotic fluid will be used to confirm results.

Urine Tests

The following are some common urine tests:

- Routine urinalysis
- Culture and sensitivity: Diagnosis urinary tract infection
- Cytology studies: Detect presence of abnormal cells from urinary tract
- Drug screening: Detects use of illegal drugs (prescription or illicit) and steroids, and monitors therapeutic drug use
- Pregnancy test: Confirms pregnancy by testing for the presence of human chorionic gonadotropin (HCG)

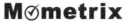

ASPECTS OF URINE REVIEWED IN ROUTINE URINALYSIS

The following are aspects of urine that are reviewed in a routine urinalysis:

- **Physical**: Color, odor, transparency, specific gravity
- **Chemical**: Looking for bacteria, blood, WBC, protein, and glucose
- **Microscopic**: Urine components (i.e., casts, cells, and crystals)

MIDSTREAM URINE COLLECTION AND MIDSTREAM CLEAN-CATCH URINE COLLECTION

Both the midstream urine collection and the midstream clean-catch urine collection methods involve an initial void into the toilet, interruption of urine flow, restart of urination into a collection container, collection of a sufficient amount of specimen, and voiding of excess urine down the toilet. The clean-catch involves cleaning of the genital area, collecting urine into a sterile container, and quickly processing it to prevent overgrowth of microorganisms, degradation of the specimen, and incorrect results.

24-HOUR URINE SPECIMEN COLLECTION

For the 24-hour urine specimen test, all of the patient's urine must be collected over the course of **24 hours**. A large collection container is provided to the patient. When a patient awakes, the first void of the morning is for the previous 24 hours and must be discarded. The next void is collected, as well as all additional voids over the next 24 hours (including the next morning's void). This specimen collection **must be kept cold**, and therefore must be refrigerated or kept on ice during the 24 hours of collection.

Processing

SPECIMEN HANDLING AND TRANSPORTING

CHAIN-OF-CUSTODY SPECIMENS

Chain-of-custody specimens are those for which a laboratory has established a documented record that shows every consecutive person in contact with the specimen from the time of collection through transfer and to the time of disposition (both internal and external contact and including date, time, and signature). This record ensures that no tampering with the specimen has occurred in order to meet legal requirements. The document must outline provisions for securing long-term storage. Chain-of-custody specimens may include specimens for blood alcohol, drugs, or crime scene testing, often including blood, urine, and DNA testing. The chain-of-custody standard operating procedure (SOP) may include labeling requirements, temperature requirements, expected timeline, packing, and transporting specifications. The person from whom the sample is obtained must be clearly identified, as well as the name of the collector and the time, date, and location of obtaining the sample. Containers in which a sample is transported should be secured with custody tape.

NEWBORN SCREENING

Newborn blood spot screening for inherited metabolic disorders should be done 24–48 hours after birth. Screening can identify up to 60 disorders, but each state sets the specific tests that will be carried out. The procedure is as follows:

1. Gather the necessary supplies and fill out the demographic portion of the collecting form.
2. Avoid touching the blood collection area of the form.
3. Wash hands, apply powder-free gloves, and select an appropriate puncture site (avoid sites with previous punctures).
4. Apply a heel warmer for 3–5 minutes and position the infant's leg lower than his or her heart.
5. Wipe the skin vigorously with an alcohol pad and allow it to completely air-dry.
6. Encircle the heel with the thumb and forefinger and gently apply pressure.
7. Puncture the heel at the medial or lateral plantar surface with a retractable heel lancet (1 mm depth and 2.5 mm length) and wipe away the first blood drop with a dry gauze square.
8. Allow a large drop to form, and then touch the first dot of the filter paper to the drop (but not the skin), allowing it to soak through. Continue until all of the dots are filled.
9. Apply a gauze pressure dressing to the wound.
10. Allow the filter paper to air-dry for 3 hours before processing.

84

SPECIMEN ASSESSMENT AND REJECTION CRITERIA

Specimens must be obtained following established protocols and in the proper tube or container with the correct additive, such as sodium citrate in a blood specimen. The specimen must be stored and/or transported in a manner appropriate to the type of specimen. **Rejection criteria** may vary according to the type of specimen and test, and specimens are generally not discarded until the ordering healthcare provider is notified. Rejection criteria may include:

- Incorrect tube or container
- Incorrect or missing requisition/order
- Specimen size insufficient for testing
- Hemolysis evident
- Specimen not correctly labeled
- Tube/container leaking or contaminated with body fluids (note: critical specimens may be salvaged after the tube/container is thoroughly cleansed with 10% hypochlorite [bleach] solution)
- Specimen contained in syringe with attached needle
- Date/collection time not noted on specimen
- Specimen too old for testing
- Specimen improperly stored/transported

ISSUES OF SPECIMEN QUALITY

Issues of specimen quality include:

- **Hemolysis**: Pink discoloration of plasma and serum because of the presence of damaged red blood cells and hemoglobin. May result from an abnormal condition, such as hemolytic anemia, or from incorrect handling. Hemolyzed samples may interfere with some tests (electrolytes, iron, enzymes), so the sample will likely need to be redrawn.
- **Quantity not sufficient (QNS)**: May occur if the volume of blood in the collection tube is insufficient for testing or if the blood-anticoagulant ratio is incorrect. Short draws may be sufficient for some tests if the specimen is not hemolyzed. With QNS, the usual solution is to obtain another specimen.
- **Clotting**: May result from maintaining a sample in a syringe with no anticoagulant for too long before transferring to a tube; from carrying out a very slow draw with a syringe that allows clotting to begin; or from failing to adequately mix the sample with the anticoagulant. If clotting occurs, a new sample must be obtained.
- **Incorrect specimen type**: If the incorrect specimen type is obtained or a specimen is obtained in a collection tube with the wrong additive, then a new specimen must be obtained in order to carry out the intended tests.

PROCEDURES TO PREVENT HEMOLYSIS

Hemolysis, rupture of red blood cells, is the most common reason laboratory specimens must be redrawn. Methods to prevent hemolysis include:

- Use a large-gauge (20–22) needle for blood draws for large veins, such as the antecubital.
- Warm the draw site to improve blood flow.
- Keep the tourniquet on for no longer than 60 seconds.
- Air-dry alcohol applied to skin prior to blood draw.
- Use partial vacuum tubes if possible.
- Avoid milking veins or capillary puncture sites.
- Avoid excessive pressure when pulling or pushing on the plunger.
- Avoid blood draws from catheters or vascular access devices.
- Ensure the volume in tubes with anticoagulant is sufficient.
- Avoid vigorous mixing or shaking of specimens.
- Invert tubes with clot activator 5 times, with anticoagulant 8–10 times, and with sodium citrate 3–4 times (coagulation tests).
- Store and transport specimens at an appropriate temperature.
- Use appropriate centrifugal speed and duration for processing samples that have clotted completely.

CLOTTING TIME CONSIDERATIONS FOR BLOOD SAMPLES

Clotting time may vary according to environmental conditions and the addition of clot activators. Clotting must be fully complete before a sample is placed in the centrifuge, or a latent formation of fibrin may clot serum. Complete clotting usually takes 30–60 minutes at temperatures of 22–25 °C (room temperature), although this time may be prolonged in samples with a high white blood cell count or in chilled samples. Clotting is also prolonged in samples of patients on anticoagulant therapy, such as heparin or warfarin. Clot activators may be added to a sample to decrease the time needed for clotting:

- Silica particles (found in serum separator tubes) and plastic red-topped tubes require 15–30 minutes.
- Thrombin tubes require about 5 minutes.

Note: 5–6 gentle inversions of a tube with clot activators, to mix it with the blood sample, are required.

SHIPPING PATIENT SAMPLES

The personnel responsible for shipping specimens must have been appropriately trained and must understand possible hazards, according to regulations by the Department of Transportation, the International Civil Aviation Organization, and the CDC. Frozen serum and plasma must be shipped in plastic tubes (not glass) with screw-on caps for security and labeled with two patient identifiers. The tubes are wrapped in absorbent material in case of leakage, secured in a container that is airtight (such as Saf-T-Pak), labeled "biohazard." This is placed inside of a Styrofoam container, for insulation, with dry ice, then this is placed in a clearly labeled secure box or temperature-controlled container. Specimens that are not frozen are similarly packaged using a specimen container, wrapped in absorbent material, placed in individual biohazard bags, and secured in a transport box of metal or plastic. The specimen may or may not be placed in a temperature-controlled container, depending on ambient temperatures.

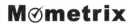

Light Considerations in Transporting Specimens and Disposition of Specimens

Most specimens are not sensitive to **light**, but some must be transported in special light-blocking containers or wrapped in aluminum foil during transport: bilirubin, carotene, red blood cell folate, serum folate, and vitamins B2, B6, B12, and C. Urine specimens for porphyrins and porphobilinogen must also be protected from light. Light-blocking amber-colored collection tubes and urine specimen containers are also available. OSHA and state regulations outline the requirements for **disposition** of blood bags and patient samples. Blood disposition must comply with OSHA's Bloodborne Pathogens Standard (29 CFR 1910.1030), which covers blood (semi-liquid, liquid, dried) in containers, in other waste products, or on items, such as sharps. As a regulated waste, the blood must be placed in a container that is closable, leak-proof, labeled (proper color-coding), and closed before removal to avoid any spillage or loss of contents during transport to the disposal site.

Specimen Processing

Properly Centrifuging a Specimen

The centrifuge needs to be evenly balanced with tubes of equal size and volume across from one another. Stoppers should always be in place to prevent aerosol. Also, be sure to allow complete clotting before centrifuging the specimen. If a specimen is not completely clotted before centrifuging, it may result in latent fibrin formations clotting the serum. Never centrifuge a specimen twice.

Settling of Blood in Anticoagulant Tubes

Blood in an anticoagulant tube will settle in this manner after being centrifuged or allowed to settle:

- The top layer will be the plasma.
- The next thin layer is the buffy coat, made of white blood cells and platelets.
- The bottom layer is red blood cells.

Aliquoting

Aliquoting a sample is done to withdraw serum or plasma from whole blood and/or to divide one sample into multiple aliquots for different tests. The individual must apply PPE, including gloves and goggles, and prepare aliquot tubes with appropriate labels. Aliquoting is done after centrifugation, with anticoagulated tubes aliquoted into plasma specimens and coagulated tubes aliquoted into serum specimens. It is necessary to place the centrifuged tubes into a rack and to avoid inverting the sample after centrifugation because this will cause remixing. A disposable pipette (never use a mouth pipette) is used to transfer each aliquot, starting from the top of the sample and working downward toward the point of separation. The aliquots are transferred to labeled tubes. As soon as an aliquot tube is filled, it must be capped. Aliquoted samples must be carefully labeled because serum and plasma are indistinguishable once they are aliquoted. Some other types of samples, such as saliva, must be mixed using a vortex mixer prior to aliquoting to ensure the sample is homogenous. Aliquots should be placed promptly in the appropriate storage, such as the refrigerator or a −20 °C or −80 °C freezer.

POUR-OFFS AND PIPETTING

During centrifugation, the denser components, such as red blood cells and cell debris, separate from the liquid components and collect at the bottom of the tube, forming the pellet. The liquid portion at the top is the supernatant, which contains plasma. Aliquoting is the process of dividing a sample into smaller portions (aliquots), such as those used for further testing. **Pour-off** is the procedure used to pour part of a sample into another container. For example, following centrifugation, all or part of the supernatant may be poured off. The tube should be handled gently and tilted slowly to pour off the supernatant, using care not to disturb the pellet. Pour-off is less precise than **pipetting**, in which pipettes are used to aliquot smaller volumes. The pipette and tip size must be appropriate for the transfer volume. Types of pipettes include air displacement and positive displacement. Different methods can be used for pipetting—forward, reverse, and repetitive—depending on the solution or compound being transferred. With all types, the volume is set before the pipette tip is inserted into the liquid and the operating button is released to draw it in. The operating button is also used to dispense the liquid.

TEMPERATURE REQUIREMENTS FOR SPECIMENS

Specimen storage is often at room temperature, which is generally based on the range found in temperature-controlled buildings: 20–25 °C. Blood bank and laboratory specimen refrigerators are maintained at 2–4 °C. Freezers are maintained at –20 °C, with some specialty freezers at –80 °C. Incubators provide for a range of temperatures, with much incubation done at 37 °C (body temperature). Samples may remain viable for different periods of time, depending on how they are stored. Some serum and plasma samples must be frozen prior to shipping. Temperature requirements depend on the type of specimen and the test.

Transport with heat block at 37 °C: Cryoglobulins, cryofibrinogen, and cold agglutinin.

The most appropriate way to **chill a specimen** is to immerse it into an ice and water slush. Ice cubes alone will not allow for adequate cooling of the specimen, and the specimen may freeze where the ice cubes touch it, resulting in possible hemolysis or breakdown of the analyte. **Transport in ice slurry and refrigerate the following samples:** adrenocorticotropic hormone (ACTH), acetone, angiotensin-converting enzyme (ACE), ammonia, blood gases, catecholamines, FFA, gastrin, glucagon, homocysteine, lactic acid, parathyroid hormone (PTH), blood pH, pyruvate, renin.

INVERTING A TUBE

A tube should be inverted if it contains an additive and if the manufacturer's instructions require it to be inverted. If the sample is in a nonadditive tube, then it does not have to be inverted. An additive tube is usually inverted 3–8 times to properly mix the additive with the blood.

PREVENTING AEROSOL FORMATION WHEN STOPPER HAS NO SAFETY FEATURE TO PREVENT AEROSOL

The stopper should be covered with 4×4-inch gauze and placed behind a safety shield to ensure the aerosol is not inhaled. Proper protective clothing should be worn as well. A safety stopper removal device may also be used.

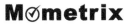

TIME CONSIDERATIONS WHEN PROCESSING SAMPLES

Specimens should be delivered to the laboratory for processing as quickly as possible and within no more than 45 minutes. STAT tests should be run first. Some tests have **time considerations** that must be followed:

- Blood gases must be processed within 20 minutes.
- Prothrombin time (PT) must be run on an unrefrigerated blood sample within 24 hours.
- Partial thromboplastin time (PTT) must be run on a room-temperature or refrigerated sample within 4 hours.

Additives also affect time considerations:

Additive	Tests	Time from collection
EDTA	Blood smear	Within 1 hour.
EDTA	CBC	Within 6 hours at room temperature and within 4 hours for micro-collection tubes. However, the sample is usually stable at room temperature for 24 hours.
EDTA	ESR	Within 4 hours at room temperature and within 12 hours if refrigerated.
EDTA	Reticulocyte count	Within 6 hours at room temperature and within 72 hours if refrigerated.
Sodium fluoride	Glucose	Within 24 hours at room temperature and within 48 hours if refrigerated.

Practice Test #1

1. Which of the following panels of tests may provide the best information about a patient with suspected liver dysfunction?

    a. BMP
    b. CMP
    c. Lipid profile
    d. Electrolyte panel

2. When collecting a blood specimen from an ambulatory patient in the home environment, the patient should be placed:

    a. In a comfortable chair
    b. Sitting at a table
    c. Recumbent or in a chair with arm supports
    d. Lying supine in bed

3. During a blood draw and collection in multiple vacuum tubes, if the third tube fails to fill, the most appropriate initial response is to:

    a. Insert the needle deeper into the vein.
    b. Discontinue the venipuncture and try a different site.
    c. Try a different vacuum tube.
    d. Call for assistance.

4. The primary focus of CLIA (1988) is to ensure that:

    a. Patients get correct laboratory results.
    b. Patients are reimbursed for errors.
    c. Patients are informed of rights.
    d. Patients are protected from injury.

5. If a patient reports a history of episodes of syncope, the most appropriate response is to:

    a. Place the patient in a recumbent position.
    b. Encourage the patient to do deep breathing and relaxation exercises.
    c. Reassure the patient that venipuncture is not painful.
    d. Provide smelling salts (ammonia inhalant).

6. When collecting a blood specimen for trace elements such as zinc, the appropriate tube type is:

    a. Plastic
    b. Metal-free
    c. Glass
    d. Stopper-free

7. When collecting a capillary blood sample after a fingerstick or heelstick, it is generally necessary to:

    a. Wipe away the first drop.
    b. Collect every drop.
    c. "Milk" the finger or heel to promote blood flow.
    d. Scrape the collector against the skin to collect the dripping blood.

8. Which of the following disinfectants may be used to prepare the venipuncture site for EtOH testing?

    a. Tincture of iodine

    b. Soap and water

    c. Isopropyl alcohol

    d. Methanol

9. All lab samples should be handled according to:

    a. Airborne precautions

    b. Contact precautions

    c. Universal precautions

    d. Standard precautions

10. Which pattern of antecubital veins is predominant in most populations?

    a. The M pattern

    b. The Y pattern

    c. The H pattern

    d. An atypical pattern

11. The primary organization/agency that accredits laboratories and publishes laboratory checklists is the:

    a. CLSI

    b. CAP

    c. FDA

    d. CDC

12. The maximum volume of blood that may be drawn from a 20 lb infant in an eight-week period is approximately:

    a. 20 mL

    b. 70 mL

    c. 100 mL

    d. 140 mL

13. A butterfly infusion set is used for venipuncture in all of the following types of patients EXCEPT:

    a. Infants

    b. Obese patients

    c. Adults with small veins

    d. Elderly patients

14. How long should the phlebotomist observe a venipuncture site for signs of excessive or persistent bleeding before applying a bandage?

    a. 1–2 seconds

    b. 3–5 seconds

    c. 5–10 seconds

    d. 10–20 seconds

15. When decanting a 24-hour urine specimen, which may splash, into a sink to a sanitary sewer, the phlebotomist should:

    a. Run water while decanting.
    b. Pour from a height of at least 6 inches.
    c. Stand as far away from the sink as possible.
    d. Wear facial protection and a fluid-proof apron.

16. If a patient has undergone bilateral mastectomies with surgeries 5 years apart, what venipuncture site should the phlebotomist select?

    a. An ankle on either side
    b. The phlebotomist should ask the physician for instructions.
    c. The arm on the side of the most recent mastectomy
    d. The arm on the side of the most distant mastectomy

17. Serum specimens can be centrifuged:

    a. Only before clotting occurs
    b. Only after clotting is completed
    c. At any stage of clotting
    d. Immediately upon receipt

18. Withdrawing blood from a VAD for noncoagulation studies requires:

    a. Waiting at least 60 minutes after a heparin flush before withdrawing blood
    b. Drawing a discard tube before withdrawing blood
    c. Flushing the VAD with preservative-free NS and drawing a discard tube first
    d. Flushing the VAD with preservative-free NS before withdrawing blood

19. One of the reasons that serum is more often used for testing than plasma is that serum contains:

    a. No clotting factors
    b. Fewer antigens
    c. More anticoagulants
    d. Fewer gases

20. When obtaining a blood specimen for coagulation tests (PT, aPTT), when is the use of a discard tube indicated?

    a. It is never indicated when obtaining a blood specimen for coagulation tests.
    b. It is always indicated when obtaining a blood specimen for coagulation tests.
    c. It is indicated whenever the coagulation tube is the first tube needed.
    d. It is indicated when a winged (butterfly) blood collection set is used and the coagulation tube is filled first.

21. A blood specimen for a CBC should be collected in a tube that contains:

    a. No additive
    b. ACD
    c. EDTA
    d. Clot activator

22. Which of the following is NOT a cause of hemolysis?

a. Failing to air dry the antiseptic
b. Using a larger-than-needed needle
c. Using a smaller-than-needed needle
d. Shaking tubes vigorously

23. For most POC pregnancy tests, when is the earliest point at which the test will be accurate?

a. Any time
b. 14 days after unprotected sex
c. 1 week after a missed period
d. 1 day after a missed period

24. If the phlebotomist tells a friend about doing a venipuncture for a famous actor who is hospitalized, this constitutes:

a. A HIPAA violation
b. Malpractice
c. Slander
d. Battery

25. If a venipuncture is performed on the basilic vein and the blood returns bright red and appears to pulse, this indicates a(n):

a. Accidental arterial draw
b. High blood pressure
c. Blood abnormality
d. Successful blood draw

26. When the phlebotomist has trouble visualizing a vein, the best approach is to:

a. Ask the patient to pump the fist.
b. Vigorously massage the area of the vein.
c. Leave the tourniquet in place for 2 minutes.
d. Ask the patient to make a fist.

27. The total blood volume of a child is approximately:

a. 65–70 mL/kg
b. 75–80 mL/kg
c. 85–105 mL/kg
d. 100–120 mL/kg

28. Which of the following specimens must be collected 2 hours after the patient has ingested a meal?

a. FBS
b. PP
c. Hgb
d. HBV

29. The most commonly used needle gauge for venipuncture is:

    a. 19
    b. 21
    c. 23
    d. 24

30. When using a portable heat block to maintain a blood specimen at body temperature, the phlebotomist should expect the heat block to hold the temperature for approximately:

    a. 5 minutes
    b. 15 minutes
    c. 60 minutes
    d. 2 hours

31. The correct angle of insertion of the needle for a venipuncture is usually:

    a. 10 degrees
    b. 20 degrees
    c. 30 degrees
    d. 45 degrees

32. The maximum number of samples or tests that can be performed each hour by an assay system is the:

    a. Input
    b. Throughput
    c. Output
    d. Continuous flow

33. When selecting an antecubital vein, priority should be given to veins in the:

    a. Lateral aspect
    b. Medial aspect
    c. Median aspect
    d. Lateral or medial aspect

34. During venipuncture, the correct position for the needle is:

    a. Bevel up at a 30-degree angle to the skin
    b. Bevel up at a 45-degree angle to the skin
    c. Bevel down at a 30-degree angle to the skin
    d. Bevel down at a 45-degree angle to the skin

35. If a patient complains of nausea after a blood draw, the most appropriate response is to:

    a. Reassure the patient that the venipuncture is completed.
    b. Give the patient an emesis basin and encourage deep breathing.
    c. Give the patient a drink of cold water.
    d. Put the patient into the flat supine position.

36. Which of the following statements regarding lumbar puncture is FALSE?

    a. The needle enters the spinal cavity.
    b. The needle enters the space between the 3rd and 4th lumbar vertebrae.
    c. The procedure poses a risk of injury to the spinal cord.
    d. The patient may experience a headache as a side effect.

37. Which type of urine specimen collection method is used in infants and small children?

  a. Clean catch
  b. Midstream clean catch
  c. Suprapubic
  d. Regular void

38. Which antiseptic is most commonly used for cleaning the venipuncture site?

  a. Chlorhexidine gluconate
  b. Povidone-iodine
  c. 70% isopropyl alcohol
  d. 90% isopropyl alcohol

39. When carrying out a rapid test for group A streptococci from a throat swab, if there is no blue control line on the dipstick at 5 minutes, the test is:

  a. Positive
  b. Negative
  c. Inconclusive
  d. Invalid

40. When venipuncture is performed in edematous tissue, the results will likely be:

  a. The same as those from normal tissue
  b. Inconclusive
  c. Contaminated with bacteria
  d. Altered

41. The best time to obtain a blood specimen for lowest cortisol level is at about:

  a. Noon
  b. Midnight
  c. 5 a.m.
  d. 8 p.m.

42. With RIDTs, both positive and negative test results are more likely to be accurate if the sample is obtained within:

  a. 1 day of the onset of symptoms
  b. 2 days of the onset of symptoms
  c. 4 days of the onset of symptoms
  d. 7 days of the onset of symptoms

43. If a patient is undergoing analysis of gastric fluids before and after a gastric stimulant, for which blood test is the phlebotomist likely to need to collect a specimen?

  a. CBC
  b. Uric acid
  c. Serum gastrin
  d. Albumin

44. Which of the following POC tests measures the volume of RBCs in a patient's blood?

 a. Hgb
 b. Hct
 c. INR
 d. Na

45. A patient with an order for blood tests has a clamped PICC line in the left arm, so the phlebotomist should draw blood from the:

 a. Right arm
 b. Left arm, distal to the PICC line
 c. Left arm, proximal to the PICC line
 d. PICC line

46. Asthma is caused by:

 a. Obstruction of the airway
 b. Inflammation of the bronchial tubes
 c. Too-rapid breathing
 d. Oxygen deficiency

47. Tests that are NOT appropriate for delivery to the lab by pneumatic tube include:

 a. Albumin
 b. Glucose
 c. Cryoglobulins
 d. Uric acid

48. *DNR* means:

 a. Do not record
 b. Does not remember
 c. Does not respond
 d. Do not resuscitate

49. The number 1 in which of the colors of an NFPA hazardous chemical label is used to indicate a substance that is reactive and normally stable but may become unstable and dangerous if heated?

 a. Blue
 b. White
 c. Yellow
 d. Red

50. Which of the following factors is likely to have the greatest effect on the results of a CBC processed within 2 hours of collection of the sample?

 a. Mealtime
 b. Mild exercise
 c. Environmental temperature
 d. Dehydration

51. A venipuncture should never be carried out proximal to a PICC line because:

  a. The blood will be diluted.
  b. The catheter may be damaged.
  c. Doing so increases the risk of thrombophlebitis.
  d. A large discard volume is required.

52. Mouth pipetting of a blood sample is:

  a. Used for skin punctures only
  b. Optional
  c. Reserved for pathologists only
  d. Prohibited

53. If a patient with rheumatoid arthritis has severe flexion contractures of both arms and hands, the best solution for selecting a venipuncture site is probably to:

  a. Ask the patient.
  b. Use the nondominant hand.
  c. Use the foot or ankle.
  d. Suggest an arterial draw.

54. If a patient must do a 72-hour stool collection for fecal fat analysis, the stool should be kept under what conditions during the collection period?

  a. At room temperature
  b. Under refrigeration
  c. Frozen in separate bags for each day
  d. In a heated container

55. The purpose of a blood transfer device is to prevent:

  a. Specimen contamination
  b. A needlestick
  c. Tube breakage
  d. Spillage

56. If the safety device on the venipuncture needle fails to activate, leaving the needle exposed, the phlebotomist should _____ to dispose of it.

  a. place the cap back on the needle
  b. bend and break the needle
  c. wrap a gauze pad around the needle
  d. carefully place the needle in the sharps container

57. Which of the following is NOT a good solution to the dealing with nonstandard shift work, such as 11 p.m. to 7 a.m.?

  a. Maintain different sleep patterns for working and nonworking days.
  b. Schedule regular naptimes.
  c. Avoid caffeinated beverages up to 6 hours before scheduled bedtime.
  d. Use room-darkening shades while sleeping.

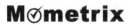

58. During a venipuncture, if the patient cries out and complains of severe pain, the most appropriate response is to:

    a. Quickly finish the draw.
    b. Ask the patient to rate the pain on a scale of 1–10.
    c. Encourage the patient to take a deep breath and relax.
    d. Immediately remove the needle.

59. If category B infectious materials must be transported out of the area for testing, specimens must not exceed:

    a. 200 mL or 200 g
    b. 300 mL or 300 g
    c. 400 mL or 400 g
    d. 500 mL or 500 g

60. When a fasting urine test is ordered for glucose testing, which of the following must be collected?

    a. Any urine specimen after a specified period of fasting
    b. The first urine specimen voided after a specified period of fasting
    c. The second urine specimen voided after a specified period of fasting
    d. The third urine specimen voided after a specified period of fasting

61. The vasovagal response is commonly known as:

    a. Allergic reaction
    b. Myocardial infarction
    c. Fainting
    d. Hematoma

62. A micro-sample is generally collected from a 9-month-old infant by:

    a. Fingerstick
    b. Scalp stick
    c. Heelstick
    d. Venipuncture

63. If peritoneal fluid is aspirated during a paracentesis and must be tested for cell counts, which type of specimen tube is indicated?

    a. EDTA
    b. Sodium fluoride
    c. Heparin
    d. Nonanticoagulant

64. In therapeutic drug monitoring, trough levels are collected:

    a. 30–60 minutes after the drug is administered
    b. To determine if the dose is toxic
    c. Prior to administration of the next dose
    d. To determine the therapeutic window

65. A used disposable needle and syringe should:
   a. Have the needle bent to prevent further use.
   b. Have the needle recapped to prevent injury.
   c. Have the needle separated from the syringe.
   d. Be placed as is in a puncture-resistant sharps container.

66. Following capillary blood collection from a heel or finger, a bandage should be applied to the collection site of patients who are:
   a. 2 years or older
   b. 1 year or older
   c. 6 months or older
   d. 3 months or older

67. If, after filling a collection tube, the phlebotomist notes blood on the outside of the tube, the correct action is to:
   a. Discard the specimen in a biohazard waste container.
   b. Wipe the tube with disinfectant and seal in a biohazard bag.
   c. Discard the specimen in a sharps container.
   d. Transport the tube to the lab in a gloved hand.

68. After collecting a blood sample, a tube containing sodium citrate as an additive should be inverted:
   a. 1–3 times
   b. 3–4 times
   c. 4–6 times
   d. 5–10 times

69. If a person's blood is type O, what plasma agglutinin is present in the person's blood?
   a. Anti-A
   b. Anti-B
   c. Anti-A and anti-B
   d. None

70. The POC test that is most accurate for monitoring heparin therapy is:
   a. PT
   b. ACT
   c. INR
   d. APTT

71. All of the following are blood gas values EXCEPT:
   a. HCO_3
   b. pH
   c. pCO_2

d. Hct

72. Which of the following actions may result in hemolysis of a specimen?
    a. Collecting a specimen from a VAD
    b. Using a 22-gauge needle for collection
    c. Leaving the tourniquet in place for 45 seconds
    d. Gently inverting the specimen

73. If a patient is heavily tattooed on both arms, from shoulders to wrists with no areas left open, the most appropriate site for venipuncture is:
    a. Any site
    b. The antecubital area with the oldest tattoos
    c. The dorsal metacarpal veins
    d. An area without solid dye

74. A biohazard sign at the entrance to the laboratory that lists the laboratory's biosafety level as 3 (BSL-3) means that the lab studies infectious agents that:
    a. Do not consistently cause human disease
    b. Pose a risk if inhaled, swallowed, or exposed to the skin
    c. Are airborne and could potentially cause lethal disease
    d. Are airborne, lethal, and for which there is no effective treatment

75. The most common patient complaint when the needle hits the median nerve during an antecubital venipuncture is:
    a. Numbness
    b. Dull aching pain
    c. Muscle twitching
    d. Severe shock-like pain

76. If a patient has made a fist for venipuncture, at what point should he or she generally be instructed to open the hand?
    a. After the needle is inserted
    b. When blood flow is established
    c. After the collection is completed
    d. After the needle is removed

77. At which of the following times are peak levels of cortisol usually obtained?
    a. In the late afternoon
    b. Around noon
    c. In the early morning
    d. At midnight

78. If a patient sitting in a chair has a generalized convulsive seizure during venipuncture, the appropriate response is to discontinue venipuncture and:
    a. Call for help to ease the patient to the floor.
    b. Restrain the patient in the chair.
    c. Support the patient in the chair and call 9-1-1.
    d. Place a tongue blade between the patient's teeth.

79. All of the following can affect GTT results EXCEPT:

   a. Aspirin
   b. Birth control pills
   c. Corticosteroids
   d. Blood pressure medications

80. The nerve most often injured with venipuncture is the _____ nerve.

   a. radial
   b. ulnar
   c. musculocutaneous
   d. median

81. When performing a venipuncture on a patient under investigation (PUI) for Ebola, the correct isolation procedure is:

   a. Contact
   b. Droplet
   c. Contact and droplet
   d. Standard, contact, and droplet plus enhanced measures

82. A sample being designated as QNS means that:

   a. The quality is not standardized.
   b. The quality is nonsterile.
   c. The quantity is not standardized.
   d. The quantity is not sufficient.

83. Black-capped collection tubes are used only for:

   a. Toxicology
   b. Lead levels
   c. Coagulation tests
   d. ESR

84. The volume of blood that a microcollection tube holds is:

   a. 0.25 mL
   b. 0.5 mL
   c. 0.75 mL
   d. 1 mL

85. When conducting the urine dipstick test, how should the dipstick be held after it is dipped into the urine sample and withdrawn?

   a. Maintained in the urine
   b. Vertically so the urine drips quickly
   c. Horizontally so the urine pools
   d. Diagonally so the urine drips slowly

86. Which of the following is an appropriate question to verify a patient's ID?

   a. "Is your name Sally Evans?"
   b. "Are you Ms. Evans? What is your birthdate?"
   c. "Ms. Evans, were you born on March 16, 1980?"
   d. "Can you tell me your name and birthdate?"

87. If less than the recommended volume necessary for blood cultures is obtained, how should the blood be distributed in the aerobic and anaerobic specimen tubes?

    a. Place equal amounts in the aerobic and anaerobic specimen tubes.
    b. Fill only the aerobic specimen tube.
    c. Fill the aerobic specimen tube completely, and place the remainder in the anaerobic tube.
    d. Fill the anaerobic specimen tube completely, and place the remainder in the aerobic tube.

88. A patient that falls and experiences a fractured hip will be treated in the:

    a. Oncology department
    b. Outpatient department
    c. Orthopedic department
    d. Obstetric department

89. If a patient in the emergency department refuses to have blood drawn but the phlebotomist does so at the physician's insistence, the phlebotomist may be charged with:

    a. Assault
    b. Negligence
    c. Malpractice
    d. Nothing

90. If a phlebotomist develops dermatitis from all types of gloves, the best solution is to:

    a. Stop wearing gloves.
    b. Double wash the hands only.
    c. Use glove liners or barrier cream.
    d. Wear gloves as briefly as possible.

91. All of the following are tests that may be performed on CSF EXCEPT:

    a. Chloride
    b. Total protein
    c. Glucose
    d. ABO

92. If a patient has severely impaired circulation in the legs and has had a recent bilateral mastectomy, the best choice for a blood draw is probably:

    a. Foot or ankle veins
    b. An artery
    c. The dominant arm
    d. The nondominant arm

93. All laboratory testing in the United States, except for research testing, is regulated by the Centers for Medicare and Medicaid Services through the:

    a. AHA
    b. CLIA
    c. CDC
    d. OIG

94. Which of the following situations introduces the most risk for error related to patient ID?
  a. Older adult patient
  b. Adolescent patient
  c. Having multiple patients in one room
  d. Outpatient

95. If an accidental arterial puncture is suspected, the correct response is to:
  a. Complete the draw and apply immediate pressure to the site.
  b. Withdraw the needle immediately and apply pressure to the site.
  c. Complete the draw and observe the puncture site for edema and bleeding.
  d. Leave the needle in place and call for help.

96. Phlebotomists are especially at risk for developing an allergic response to:
  a. Latex
  b. Alcohol
  c. Plastic
  d. Nitrile

97. The peak time for most drugs after intramuscular injection is approximately _____, which is relevant for timing sample collection for therapeutic drug monitoring.
  a. 30 minutes
  b. 60 minutes
  c. 90 minutes
  d. 2 hours

98. Which of the following tests is used to assess thyroid function?
  a. GH
  b. GTT
  c. ADH
  d. TSH

99. Which of the following statements regarding warming of the injection site is FALSE?
  a. Warming the site is necessary for collecting blood gas specimens.
  b. Warming is required for fingersticks in patients with cold hands.
  c. Warming significantly alters results of routine analyte testing.
  d. Warming is recommended for heelstick procedures in infants.

100. The _____ plane divides the body into anterior and posterior sections.
  a. sagittal
  b. midsagittal
  c. transverse
  d. coronal

101. Which of the following tests requires a timed specimen?
  a. CBC
  b. Uric acid
  c. Blood culture
  d. Cortisol

102. If, after obtaining a blood sample, a phlebotomist accidentally experiences a needlestick that does not draw blood, the phlebotomist should:

a. Wash the site with soap and water and take no further action.
b. Wipe the site with an alcohol swab and verify that there is no bleeding.
c. Wash the site with soap and water and report the incident.
d. Flush the site with running water for 20 minutes and report the incident.

103. When collecting a specimen from a patient in a long-term-care facility, the first thing the phlebotomist should do is to:

a. Knock on the patient's door.
b. Check in at the nursing station.
c. Contact the patient prior to arrival.
d. Enter the patient's room.

104. If a specimen must be chilled, the best method is to:

a. Place it in a water-and-ice mixture.
b. Cover it with ice.
c. Refrigerate it.
d. Place it in dry ice.

105. At room temperature, complete clotting usually occurs within:

a. 10–15 minutes
b. 15–30 minutes
c. 30–60 minutes
d. 60–90 minutes

106. If CSF is collected in four numbered containers, the first tube is used for:

a. Microbiology studies
b. Cell count and differential
c. Cytology and special tests
d. Chemistry and immunology tests

107. The throat is also known as the:

a. Trachea
b. Larynx
c. Pharynx
d. Epiglottis

108. The most common reason for rejecting a specimen for chemistry is:

a. An underfilled tube
b. An overfilled tube
c. Clotting
d. Hemolysis

109. If a child weighs 30 pounds, the maximum volume of blood that can be drawn in a 24-hr period is approximately:

 a. 25 mL
 b. 50 mL
 c. 100 mL
 d. 200 mL

110. Strenuous exercise may increase values of which of the following tests for more than 24 hours?

 a. Aldosterone
 b. Lactic acid
 c. Albumin
 d. Lactic dehydrogenase (LD)

111. Plasma specimens for ammonia levels should be separated from the blood cells and tested within:

 a. 15 minutes
 b. 30 minutes
 c. 60 minutes
 d. 4 hours

112. Control runs of automated systems should be carried out:

 a. Monthly
 b. Weekly
 c. At the end of each day
 d. At the beginning of each day

113. Serous fluid may be obtained from all of the following EXCEPT:

 a. Peritoneal cavity
 b. Pleural cavity
 c. Pericardial cavity
 d. Spinal cavity

114. The additive that is most effective at preserving coagulation factors is:

 a. Potassium oxalate
 b. Lithium heparin
 c. Na_2EDTA
 d. Sodium citrate

115. When collecting a blood specimen from a patient in an isolation room, the phlebotomist should place the collection tray:

 a. At the nurse's station or another secured area
 b. On a table or chair outside of the room
 c. On a table or chair immediately inside the room
 d. On the bedside table

116. If a patient had a right mastectomy 6 months ago, blood may be drawn from the:

    a. Left arm
    b. Left or right ankle
    c. Right arm—distal area only
    d. Left or right arm

117. Which of the following is NOT a characteristic of a safety feature for a venipuncture needle?

    a. Activation is from behind the needle.
    b. Activation requires one hand only.
    c. Needle may be detached.
    d. Needle is permanent contained.

118. If a blood specimen is to be obtained for the trough level of a drug, the best time to draw the blood is usually:

    a. 15 minutes before the next scheduled dose
    b. 30 minutes before the next scheduled dose
    c. 60 minutes before the next scheduled dose
    d. 2 hours after the last scheduled dose

119. The infections most commonly transmitted through needlestick and sharp injuries are:

    a. HBV, HCV, and HIV
    b. HBV, HIV, and HZV
    c. HIV, syphilis, and CMV
    d. HBV, HB, and HZV

120. Which of the following tests requires that the specimen be chilled?

    a. Potassium
    b. CBC
    c. Uric acid
    d. Lactic acid

Answer Key and Explanations for Test #1

1. B: The CMP (comprehensive metabolic panel) contains the tests found in the BMP (basic metabolic panel)—blood urea nitrogen (BUN), Ca, CO_2, Cl, creatinine, glucose, K, and Na—along with additional tests that provide information about liver function (albumin, ALP, AST, bilirubin, and total protein). While these are fewer specific tests than found in the liver function panel, the CMP is often used to screen for liver dysfunction, and further testing may be ordered based on the results of the CMP.

2. C: When collecting a blood specimen from an ambulatory patient in the home environment, the patient should be placed recumbent or in a chair with arm supports. Venipuncture should never be carried out with the patient sitting in a chair without arm rests because, if the patient faints, the patient could easily fall out of the chair and suffer injuries. If no chair with arms is available, blood can be drawn with the patient lying in bed or on a sofa.

3. C: During a blood draw and collection in multiple vacuum tubes, if the third tube fails to fill, the most appropriate initial response is to try a different vacuum tube. Tubes sometimes lose their vacuum. If the new tube also does not fill, then the phlebotomist should check to make sure that the entire bevel of the needle is completely under the skin. If a new tube does not solve the problem and the needle is in the correct place, the venipuncture may need to be discontinued and a new site tried.

4. A: The primary focus of CLIA (Clinical Laboratory Improvement Amendments) (1988) is to ensure that patients get correct laboratory results through requiring that laboratories meet quality standards. Laboratories are required to be certified by state authorities and by CMS (Center for Medicare and Medicaid Services). The three agencies that are responsible for CLIA are:

- FDA (Food and Drug Administration) categorizes tests and develops rules
- CMS issues certificates, inspects facilities, publishes rules, and monitors lab performance
- CDC (Centers for Disease Control and Prevention) provides research, develops information, and manages the advisory committee (CLIAC)

5. A: If a patient reports a history of episodes of syncope, the most appropriate response is to place the patient in a recumbent position, either lying flat or reclining in a chair, so that he or she does not fall or experience injury if an episode of syncope occurs. Syncope is fainting that occurs with a sudden drop in blood pressure, and is sometimes associated with stress or fear. Patients who are fearful of needles or the sight of blood are especially at risk for syncope during venipuncture.

6. B: When collecting a blood specimen for trace elements, such as zinc, selenium, or mercury, the appropriate tube type is metal-free. These are specialty tubes designed so that they do not contaminate the sample with trace elements (including, but not limited to, metals) that are typically found in glass and plastic containers. These tubes usually have royal-blue tops and are available with EDTA or heparin, or they are free of additives. Samples for lead testing are collected in tan-topped tubes containing K_2EDTA.

7. A: When collecting a capillary blood sample after a fingerstick or heelstick, it is generally necessary to wipe away the first drop with a gauze pad because this first drop is likely to be contaminated and may contain some alcohol from the antiseptic, which may cause hemolysis or prevent the blood from forming drops. However, some point-of-care (POC) testing devices, such as those for glucose testing, recommend using the first drop, making them exceptions to the rule.

8. B: During blood alcohol (ethanol, or EtOH) testing, regular soap and water may be used to clean the venipuncture site if a non-alcohol disinfectant such as povidone-iodine or aqueous benzalkonium chloride is not available. Disinfectants that contain alcohol, such as tincture of iodine, isopropyl alcohol, or methanol, should not be used because they may compromise test results.

9. D: All lab samples should be handled according to standard precautions, which combine universal precautions and body substance isolation, because of the concern that not all infectious processes are obvious or identified. With body substance isolation, gloves must be worn for all contact with blood, body fluids, and any moist body surface such as mucous membranes. With universal precautions, all blood and body fluids are considered potentially infectious. Standard precautions also require respiratory hygiene/cough etiquette.

10. C: The pattern of antecubital veins that is predominant in most populations is the H pattern, also known as the N pattern. The veins that are most prominent in the H pattern include the cephalic, median cubital, and basilic veins. The veins that are most prominent in the M pattern, also known as the Y pattern, include the cephalic, median cephalic, median basilic, and basilic veins. Although these two patterns are the most common, some patients have atypical patterns of veins rather than the H or M configuration.

11. B: The primary organization/agency that accredits laboratories and publishes laboratory checklists is the College of American Pathologists (CAP). CAP accreditation is voluntary, but to qualify, labs must meet standards established in the checklists. CAP produces checklists utilizing standards produced by the Clinical Laboratory Standards Institute (CLSI). Laboratories that are CAP accredited are usually exempt from inspection by government agencies because they are considered to be in compliance with requirements established by the Clinical Laboratory Improvement Act.

12. B: The maximum volume of blood that may be drawn from a 20 lb infant in an eight-week period is approximately 70 mL. CLSI regulations recommend that no more than 10% of total blood volume be drawn from a pediatric patient over an eight-week period. Using an estimate of 75–80 mL/kg (a typical blood volume for an infant), this patient's total volume can be calculated as follows:

$$20 \text{ lb} \times \frac{1 \text{ kg}}{2.2 \text{ lb}} = 9.1 \text{ kg}$$

$$9.1 \text{ kg} \times 75 \frac{\text{mL}}{\text{kg}} = 683 \text{ mL}; \quad 9.1 \text{ kg} \times 80 \frac{\text{mL}}{\text{kg}} = 728 \text{ mL}$$

Therefore, the maximum allowable amount of blood to be drawn in this timeframe is 68–73 mL, or approximately 70 mL.

13. B: A butterfly infusion set is used for venipuncture in patients with small, fragile veins, such as the elderly, infants and small children, and adults with small antecubital veins. A butterfly set is not routinely used in obese patients.

14. C: The phlebotomist should observe a venipuncture site for 5–10 seconds for signs of excessive or persistent bleeding before applying a gauze pressure bandage. If there is bleeding, direct pressure should be applied until the bleeding is stopped and then the pressure dressing is applied. The patient should avoid exposing the site to direct pressure (such as that from a purse strap) or exertion for the next several hours to avoid reopening the wound and causing bleeding.

15. D: When decanting a 24-hour urine specimen, which may splash, into a sink to a sanitary sewer, the phlebotomist should wear facial protection and a fluid-proof apron in addition to the standard PPE (gloves, lab coat). The phlebotomist should stand close to the sink and pour close to the drain opening. Water should not be running while decanting because this increases the risk of splashing, but copious amounts of water should be run after the decanting is completed.

16. B: If a patient has undergone bilateral mastectomies with surgeries 5 years apart, the phlebotomist should ask the physician for instructions regarding the appropriate site. If policy precludes the use of the lower extremities, the venipuncture site is usually the arm on the side with the most distant mastectomy because the healing is more advanced. However, placing a tourniquet on the side of a mastectomy increases the risk of lymphedema, and the impaired lymphatic filtering and drainage also increases the risk of infection.

17. B: Serum specimens can be centrifuged only after clotting is completed. All specimens for tests carried out on serum or plasma must be centrifuged to separate the liquid from the cellular portions of the blood. However, plasma specimens that are collected in tubes with anticoagulant can be centrifuged immediately. It is important to avoid recentrifugation because this may result in hemolysis and can alter the testing results.

18. C: Withdrawing blood from a vascular access device (VAD) for coagulation studies requires flushing the VAD lock with 5–10 mL preservative-free normal saline (NS) and drawing a discard tube, equal to two times the dead space, before drawing the sample. For most central lines, 5 mL is adequate as the discard volume, although this may vary so the discard volume needed should always be verified. For coagulation studies, typically a discard volume of six times the dead space is recommended, although if drawing blood from a saline lock, a discard volume of two times the dead space is adequate. After the specimen is obtained, the VAD is again flushed with 5–10 mL of preservative-free NS.

19. A: One of the reasons that serum is more often used for testing than plasma is that serum does not contain clotting factors (e.g., fibrinogen), which could interfere with some tests. While plasma may be administered as transfusions because it contains the clotting factors needed by transfusion recipients, serum is more commonly used for testing. In some cases, a test can be done with either plasma or serum; there may be different reference ranges for the two sample types. If a patient is to have serial testing for monitoring purposes, it is important to use the same sample type every time to avoid apparent changes due to the inconsistency.

20. D: When obtaining a blood specimen for coagulation tests (PT, aPTT), the use of a discard tube is indicated when a winged (butterfly) blood collection set is used and the coagulation tube is filled first. At one time, it was standard procedure to obtain a discard tube of 5 mL of blood when the coagulation tube was the first tube to be filled, but studies have indicated that this is not necessary when using a straight needle. However, when using a winged (butterfly) needle, the discard tube is collected in order to prime the tubing so that the correct ratio of blood to anticoagulant is maintained.

21. C: A blood specimen for a CBC should be collected in a tube that contains EDTA (an anticoagulant). The CBC is performed on whole blood. The evacuated collection tube is lavender-capped and should be inverted at least 8 times after the specimen is collected to ensure that the sample is adequately anticoagulated because even small clots render the specimen unusable. The CBC includes Hgb (hemoglobin), Hct (hematocrit), RBC, RBC indices, WBC count and differential, and platelet count.

22. B: Using a larger-than-needed needle does not result in hemolysis (rupturing of RBCs), but using too small of a needle may. Other causes of hemolysis include failing to air dry the antiseptic before venipuncture, withdrawing blood from the area of a hematoma, shaking the collection tube instead of inverting to mix the blood with additive, rapidly emptying blood from a syringe into a collection tube, and withdrawing the plunger on a syringe too forcefully.

23. D: For most point-of-care (POC) pregnancy tests, the earliest time at which the test will be accurate is 1 day after a missed period. If the patient is unsure about when her period is due, then the test can be taken 21 days after unprotected sex. Some newer tests are now able to detect pregnancy even before a missed period. However, testing too early can sometimes produce a false negative, so tests taken after a missed period are usually more accurate. Testing is carried out with a urine sample.

24. A: If the phlebotomist tells a friend about doing a venipuncture for a famous actor who is hospitalized, this constitutes a Health Insurance Portability and Accountability Act of 1996 (HIPAA) violation. No protected health information, including the fact that the person was hospitalized or having tests, can be divulged without written authorization. In fact, this information must not be shared with coworkers either unless they are involved in the patient's care and have a need to know.

25. A: If venipuncture is done on the basilic vein and the blood returns bright red and pulsing, this indicates an accidental arterial draw. Venous blood should be dark purplish red, not bright red, which indicates oxygenated blood. Pulsing is characteristic of arterial blood. The basilic vein lies very close to the brachial artery. The most common reason for accidental arterial draw is deep probing for a vein. Hematoma and compression of the nerves, sometimes resulting in permanent injury, can occur if the arterial draw is not identified and adequate pressure applied to stop bleeding.

26. D: When having trouble visualizing a vein, the best approach is to ask the patient to make a fist but to avoid having them pump the fist because this may result in hemoconcentration and can affect the test results, especially that of potassium. The fist should be released as soon as blood begins to flow into the collection tube. Vigorously massaging the vein or leaving the tourniquet in place for more than 60 seconds can also cause hemoconcentration.

27. B: The total blood volume of a child is approximately 75–80 mL/kg. Blood volume is greater in a premature neonate, ranging from 89 mL/kg to approximately 105 mL/kg. The volume of blood in a full-term neonate is approximately 82–86 mL/kg. Blood volume peaks at approximately 4 weeks of age and then decreases over the next few months. The total volume of blood in an adult is typically 65–70 mL/kg.

28. B: A postprandial (PP) specimen is collected 2 hours after ingestion of a meal. Fasting blood sugar (FBS) testing occurs after the patient has fasted for 12 hours. Hgb, or hemoglobin, may be collected regardless of meals. HBV is hepatitis B virus.

29. B: The most commonly used needle gauge for venipuncture is 21. The size of the needle decreases with increasing numbers, so 21-gauge is larger than 23-gauge. Using a needle larger than 21-gauge should be avoided because it may result in extra pain and has few benefits. If the patient's veins are smaller, a 23-gauge needle may be used, but smaller gauges may increase the risk of hemolysis and also increase the time needed to collect a specimen.

30. B: When using a portable heat block to maintain a blood specimen at body temperature, the phlebotomist should expect the heat block to hold the temperature for approximately 15 minutes.

Typically, the specimen tube should also be prewarmed to body temperature or 37 °C (98.6 °F). The specimen should be transported to the lab as soon as possible and transferred to a heating device that will maintain the appropriate temperature.

31. C: The correct angle of insertion of the needle for a venipuncture is usually 30 degrees, per CLSI guidelines. If the angle is too narrow (10–20 degrees), the needle may not penetrate the vein and may enter only the subcutaneous tissue. If the angle is too steep (>30 degrees), the needle may go through the vein. However, each patient should be assessed individually. If a patient is extremely thin or is obese, the angle may need to be adjusted slightly to compensate.

32. B: The maximum number of samples or tests that can be performed each hour by an assay system is the throughput. The throughput is calculated keeping the required dwell times in mind. The throughput varies from one type of equipment to another. Throughput is one of the aspects to consider when determining turnaround time for a laboratory. Turnaround time is a key element of quality control performance. Generally, the turnaround time for the most common laboratory tests should be less than 60 minutes.

33. C: When selecting an antecubital vein, priority should be given to veins in the median (middle) aspect. These include the median vein and the lateral aspect of the median cubital vein. If these are not satisfactory, the next to consider are the veins in the lateral (outer) aspect, including the cephalic vein and the accessory cephalic vein, although there is increased risk of injury to the lateral nerve. The last to consider are the veins in the medial (inner) aspect. These include the basilic vein and the medial aspect of the median cubital vein. Venipuncture in these veins poses increased risk of injury to the brachial artery and median antebrachial cutaneous nerves.

34. A: During venipuncture, the correct position for the needle is bevel up at a 30-degree angle to the skin. Inserting at too steep of an angle can result in the needle being inserted too far, and this increases the risk of damage to nerves and arteries. However, if the needle is not inserted deeply enough, it may miss the vein. This may occur in patients whose veins are especially deep or in patients who are markedly obese.

35. B: If a patient complains of nausea after a blood draw, the most appropriate response is to give the patient an emesis basin (because nausea often leads to vomiting) and encourage deep breathing because this sometimes eases nausea. A cool, damp cloth may also be applied to the patient's forehead. In most cases, nausea subsides within a few moments, but first-aid personnel should be notified. If the patient is lying flat and supine, he or she should be turned to one side to avoid aspiration if vomiting occurs.

36. C: Because the spinal cord ends at the first lumbar vertebra, lumbar puncture does not present a risk of spinal cord injury. The physician inserts the needle into the spinal cavity at the space between the 3rd and 4th lumbar vertebrae. The patient may experience a headache as a result of the drop in pressure around the brain caused by the removal of cerebrospinal fluid.

37. C: A suprapubic specimen may be collected for infants or small children to ensure that the sample is not contaminated; this method consists of inserting a needle through the body wall and into the bladder, then collecting urine in a syringe. The clean catch and midstream clean catch methods are used for adults to ensure an uncontaminated specimen. For a regular void specimen, urine is simply collected in a wide-mouth container.

38. C: The antiseptic that is most commonly used for cleaning the venipuncture site is 70% isopropyl alcohol, which is more effective at destroying pathogens than 90% isopropyl alcohol is. Povidone-iodine may also be used, and is generally used for blood alcohol testing, but it must be removed from the skin after the venipuncture. Chlorhexidine gluconate may be used as an antiseptic as well; it is sometimes mixed with 67% isopropyl alcohol.

39. D: When carrying out a rapid test for group A streptococci from a throat swab, if there is no blue control line on the dipstick at 5 minutes, the test is invalid, possibly because the dipstick is outdated. For the test, a tube is filled with three drops each of reagents A and B and the swab is placed into the tube for 1 minute and rotated at least five times before removal. The dipstick is then placed in the tube for 5 minutes. The blue control line must appear within 5 minutes for a valid test. A positive finding is a pink or purple test line.

40. D: When venipuncture is performed in edematous tissue, the results will likely be altered because the sample may contain tissue fluid. Additionally, veins are often harder to locate in edematous tissue, and bleeding may persist longer than usual. Edematous tissue is more prone to injury from the tourniquet because the tissue is stretched. Whenever possible, a nonedematous site should be used for venipuncture. If the edema is because an IV has infiltrated, the phlebotomist must notify the nurse immediately.

41. B: The best time to obtain a blood specimen for lowest cortisol level is at about midnight. Increased levels of cortisol indicate adrenal hyperfunction and Cushing syndrome, while decreased levels indicate hypofunction and Addison's disease. Cortisol levels exhibit diurnal variation, usually peaking in the early morning (about 8 a.m.) and reaching the lowest level around midnight, so multiple tests may be ordered at different times. If cortisol tests are abnormal, additional tests are usually ordered to confirm a diagnosis.

42. C: With rapid influenza diagnostic tests (RIDTs), both positive and negative test results are more likely to be accurate if the sample is obtained within 4 days of the onset of symptoms. Both false negatives and false positives may occur, although false negatives are more common than false positives. Various tests are available. Some differentiate between influenza A and influenza B, and others do not. Different types of specimens (e.g., nasal, throat swab) are required, depending on the manufacturer.

43. C: If a patient is undergoing analysis of gastric fluids before and after a gastric stimulant, the blood test that the phlebotomist is likely to need to collect a specimen for is serum gastrin, which evaluates gastric production. The serum is collected in a red- or gray-topped tube. Gastric fluid analysis and serum gastrin are tested to help diagnose chronic gastritis, chronic renal failure, gastric and duodenal ulcers, gastric carcinoma, G-cell hyperplasia, pernicious anemia, pyloric obstruction, and hyperparathyroidism.

44. B: Hematocrit (Hct), also called packed cell volume (PCV), measures the volume of RBCs in a patient's blood. A small sample of anticoagulated blood is centrifuged; the results reflect the percentage of cells to liquid. The normal hematocrit value varies according to gender and age:

Age	Male	Female
0 to 1 week	46–68	46–68
1 to 2 months	32–54	32–54
3 months to 5 years	31–43	31–43
6 to 8 years	33–41	33–41
15 to adult	38–51	33–45
Older adult	36–52	34–46

45. A: A patient with an order for blood tests has a clamped peripherally inserted central catheter (PICC) line in the left arm, so the phlebotomist should draw blood from the right arm. Drawing blood from a vascular access device, such as a PICC line, is outside of the scope of practice of the phlebotomist; however, the phlebotomist may provide necessary collection tubes to a nurse or physician who accesses the PICC line and may transport the tubes. If a PICC line is in one arm, the opposite arm should be used for venipuncture if possible.

46. A: Asthma is caused by obstruction of the airway due to inflammation. Bronchitis is caused by inflammation of the bronchial tubes. Hyperventilation is characterized by rapid breathing resulting in a loss of carbon dioxide. Hypoxia is caused by oxygen deficiency.

47. C: Tests that are not appropriate for delivery to the lab by pneumatic tube include those in which damage to the cell membrane may affect the test results, such as lactate dehydrogenase, potassium, hemoglobin (plasma), and acid phosphatase. Additionally, samples that must be kept at body temperature, such as cryoglobulins and cold agglutinins, should not be transported by pneumatic tube. Pneumatic tubes are one of the most common methods used to transport specimens to laboratories.

48. D: *DNR* stands for "do not resuscitate." When patients are admitted to the hospital, they are usually asked if they want to be resuscitated in the event of a cardiac arrest or cessation of breathing. If patients indicate that they do not want resuscitation, then the DNR order is entered into the patient's records so that appropriate healthcare providers are aware of the patient's wishes. If no DNR order is present, then extraordinary means, such as intubation and ventilation, may be used to sustain life.

49. C: Most hazardous materials come with NFPA (National Fire Protection Association) warning labels made up of color-coded diamonds to indicate the type of risk, each with a rating from 0 (no risk) to 4 (extreme risk):

- Yellow: instability hazard
- Blue: health hazard
- Red: fire hazard
- White: other hazard (lists specific hazards, if any; does not use 0–4 rating)

In the instability (yellow) diamond, 0 indicates normally stable, 1 indicates unstable if heated, 2 indicates the substance may undergo a violent chemical reaction, 3 indicates a severe risk of explosion under certain conditions, and 4 indicates an extreme hazard that may detonate or explode at normal temperatures.

50. D: The factor that is likely to have the greatest effect on the CBC (complete blood count) is dehydration because it decreases the fluid portion of the blood, resulting in hemoconcentration. This causes the relative RBC count and the hematocrit to increase. Aerobic exercise has been shown to decrease WBC and neutrophil counts. Environmental temperature may alter some values in a CBC (RBC, Hct, MCV, MCH, and MCHC) if the sample is stored at room temperature for extended periods of time (≥24 hours).

51. B: A venipuncture should never be carried out proximal to a peripherally inserted central catheter (PICC) line because the catheter may be damaged when the tourniquet is applied or the needle is inserted and could even break, causing fragments to migrate. If possible, the arm with a PICC line should be avoided for blood draws; however, if it is absolutely necessary, the tourniquet must be placed and the venipuncture performed distal to the PICC line.

52. D: Mouth pipetting, which involves sucking a laboratory specimen into an open-ended tube, was once common practice in laboratories, but the practice was generally stopped in the 1970s when mechanical pipettes became available. However, mouth pipetting is still commonly used in developing nations where medical supplies are scarce and equipment is often outdated, so phlebotomists who work overseas should be aware that the practice puts them at high risk of disease and should never be utilized.

53. A: If a patient with rheumatoid arthritis has severe flexion contractures of both arms and hands, the best solution for selecting a venipuncture site is probably to ask the patient, who likely has had experience with blood draws and knows which sites are most easily accessed. A winged infusion set with 12-inch tubing may be the best choice because it allows for more flexibility in accessing veins when the patient is unable to extend or rotate a limb.

54. B: If a patient must do a 72-hour stool collection for fecal fat analysis, the stool should be kept under refrigeration during the collection period. The patient is provided a large gallon container with a lid and written and verbal instructions. The patient should be cautioned to avoid contaminating the stool specimen with urine, which may alter the test results. One method of collecting the stool is to place plastic wrap securely over the back half of the toilet bowl. Special collection devices are also available.

55. B: The purpose of a blood transfer device is to prevent a needlestick. The blood transfer device was devised when OSHA required that safety needles be used when collecting blood specimens. These needles cannot be used to inject blood into a collection tube, so the safety needle is removed and the transfer device, which contains a small needle inside, is attached to the luer of the syringe. The collection tube is then inserted into the transfer device and the blood is transferred when the needle penetrates the cap.

56. D: If the safety device on the venipuncture needle fails to activate, leaving the needle exposed, the phlebotomist should dispose of it by carefully placing the needle and attached tube holder in the sharps container. Needles should never be bent, broken, recapped, or wrapped, as these actions may result in needlestick injuries. The phlebotomist should report the failure of the safety device to a supervisor so that other needle supplies can be evaluated.

57. A: Because it is difficult for the body to adjust to different sleep times, a person working a nontraditional shift, such as 11 p.m. to 7 a.m., should try to maintain the same sleep patterns for both working and nonworking days. Additionally, scheduling a short nap and avoiding caffeinated beverages for at least 6 hours before scheduled bedtime may help the person get adequate sleep. Keeping the bedroom dark, such as with room-darkening shades, during sleeping hours may also help.

58. D: During a venipuncture, if the patient cries out and complains of severe pain, the most appropriate response is to immediately remove the needle even if it is in the middle of a draw. Severe pain may be an indication of damage to a nerve. Symptoms of nerve injury may additionally include shooting pain or shock-like electrical pain, tingling, numbness, or tremor in the limb. If the blood draw must still be done, another site (such as the opposite arm) must be selected. The injury must be documented, and the ordering healthcare provider must be notified.

59. D: If category B infectious materials must be transported out of the area for testing, specimens must not exceed 500 mL or 500 g. The sample must be triple wrapped. The inner container must be watertight and have a screw-on cap. This container must be wrapped in absorbent material and placed in a leakproof bag, which is then placed in a third outer container made of rigid material (wood, metal, plastic, or corrugated fiberboard). Ice or dry ice is placed around the secondary container. The outer container must be leakproof if ice is used.

60. C: When a fasting urine test is ordered for glucose testing, the second urine specimen voided after a specified period of fasting, usually 8 hours, should be collected. The first specimen, which is affected by food eaten before the fasting period, is discarded. If a first-voiding specimen is ordered, it is usually collected first thing in the morning after approximately 8 hours of sleep. First-voiding specimens are usually more concentrated than subsequent voids. Random urine specimens may be obtained at any time.

61. C: The vasovagal response is fainting or loss of consciousness due to a nervous system response to abrupt pain or trauma, and may occur during arterial puncture. A hematoma is the appearance of swelling or a blood mass during or following venipuncture. Myocardial infarction is also known as heart attack.

62. C: Blood from infants under one year of age is collected by heelstick (lateral areas), as the child's veins are generally too small for venipuncture. Once a site is selected, it should be thoroughly cleansed with antiseptic (usually 70% isopropyl alcohol) and air-dried completely. The best choice of lancet is an automated one with a controlled length of lancet to ensure that it does not insert more than 2 mm, which may result in damage to the bone.

63. A: When peritoneal fluid is aspirated during a paracentesis and must be tested for cell counts, the type of specimen tube that is indicated is EDTA. A sterile heparinized tube is used for cultures, a heparin or sodium fluoride tube is for chemistries, and a nonanticoagulant tube is for biochemical tests. Serous fluid is usually pale yellow in appearance and may include pericardial fluid that surrounds the heart, pleural fluid from the space around the lungs, and peritoneal fluid from the abdominal cavity.

64. C: Trough levels are collected when the serum concentration of the drug is at its lowest level, usually just prior to administration of the next dose. Peak levels are collected when the serum concentration is highest, usually 30–60 minutes after drug administration. If the peak level is above the toxic threshold, the dose is toxic and must be decreased. The therapeutic window is the range of blood concentrations of the drug between the minimum effective concentration and the toxic concentration.

65. D: A used disposable needle and syringe should be placed as-is in a puncture-resistant sharps container. Needles should not be bent, recapped, or separated from the syringe because any handling of the needle introduces the risk of a needlestick injury. Needles and syringes should be placed in the sharps container immediately after use whenever possible. Sharps that are nondisposable must be placed in a hard-walled container and taken to the processing area to be decontaminated.

66. A: Following capillary blood collection from a heel or finger, a bandage should be applied to the collection site of patients who are 2 years old or older. Newborns and infants younger than 2 should not be bandaged for two reasons. First, the bandage may pose a choking risk because of the child's tendency to put things in the mouth. Second, the skin is too friable and may become irritated or tear when the bandage is removed.

67. B: While wearing gloves and using care to not allow the collection tube to come into contact with any items on the blood collection tray, the phlebotomist should carefully wipe all blood from the collection tube with a disinfectant and then seal the collection tube in a biohazard bag prior to placing it on the blood collection tray for transport to the laboratory. The gloves should be disposed of in the hazardous waste container.

68. B: After collecting a blood sample, a tube containing sodium citrate as an additive should be inverted 3–4 times rather than the 5–10 times required of other additives. Sodium citrate is an anticoagulant that binds to calcium, preventing blood clotting. Sodium citrate is preferred for coagulation tests (partial thromboplastin time [PTT] and activated partial thromboplastin time [aPTT]) because it best preserves coagulation factors. Tubes that contain sodium citrate have light-blue colored stoppers or black stoppers in special tubes used for the erythrocyte sedimentation rate. Shaking or inverting too much may activate the platelets, resulting in a shortened coagulation time.

69. C: Blood type is determined by the presence or absence of antigens on the red blood cells (RBCs). If a person's blood is type A, there are A antigens on the RBCs, and the plasma agglutinin (antibody) that is present in the person's blood is anti-B. Type B blood has B antigens on the RBCs and anti-A agglutinins in the plasma. Type O blood has no antigens on the RBCs but both anti-A and anti-B agglutinins in the plasma. Individuals with type O blood, specifically O-negative blood, are considered universal donors due to their lack of antigens, making the blood less likely to be rejected or result in a transfusion reaction.

70. B: Even though aPTT is more commonly used to monitor heparin, the test that is most accurate is activated clotting time (ACT). Automated ACT analyzers measure how long it takes a blood sample to clot when activators are added to activate the clotting factors. This helps to determine how the body will respond to heparin and is more accurate than aPTT, especially if the patient is receiving high doses of heparin. The normal value for ACT may vary according to the equipment used, but it is generally 70–120 seconds. The therapeutic value is generally 150–600 seconds.

71. D: Although values for hematocrit (Hct) are often measured by blood gas analyzers, Hct is not a blood gas value; it is part of a complete blood count (CBC). Bicarbonate (HCO_3), pH, and partial pressure of carbon dioxide (pCO_2) are all blood gas values.

72. A: Collecting a specimen from a vascular access device (VAD) may result in hemolysis of a specimen. A specimen should also not be collected during an intravenous (IV) line start. Additional precautions include ensuring that the needle is secure, avoiding forcibly pulling on a plunger to withdraw blood or forcefully transferring blood from a syringe into a tube, discontinuing a sluggish draw, avoiding the use of 25-gauge needles, limiting tourniquet use to 60 seconds, and avoiding shaking or vigorously mixing specimens.

73. C: If a patient is heavily tattooed on both arms, from shoulders to wrists with no areas left open, the most appropriate site for venipuncture is the dorsal metacarpal veins. Tattooed areas should be avoided if possible because they may harbor infection (if done recently) and may mask signs of inflammation or bruising. If it is necessary to draw blood from a tattooed area, it is important to try to find an area that is open and free of dye, especially solid-dyed areas.

74. C: A biohazard sign at the entrance to the laboratory that lists the laboratory's biosafety level as 3 (BSL-3) means that the lab handles infectious agents that are airborne and could potentially cause lethal disease, such as COVID-19 and *Mycobacterium tuberculosis*. The biosafety levels are:

- BSL-1: Infectious agents do not consistently cause disease.
- BSL-2: Infectious agents pose a risk if inhaled, swallowed, or exposed to the skin.

- BSL-3: Infectious agents are airborne and could potentially cause lethal disease.
- BSL-4: Infectious agents are airborne, lethal, and no effective treatment is available.

75. D: The most common patient complaint when the needle hits the median nerve during an antecubital venipuncture is severe shock-like pain. If this occurs, the initial response should be to immediately remove the needle and apply pressure because continuing with the venipuncture may result in permanent damage to the nerve. The pain usually resolves within a few hours, but if the nerve is damaged, the patient may develop permanent pain and weakness, including complex regional pain syndrome.

76. B: If a patient has made a fist for venipuncture, the point at which he or she should generally be instructed to open the hand is when blood flow is established. The purpose of making a fist is to increase the pressure in the veins and thus their visibility. The patient should be cautioned to avoid pumping the fist, which can increase potassium levels. The hand may remain clenched during collection if the vein appears that it may collapse if the fist is unclenched.

77. C: Peak levels of cortisol are usually obtained in the early morning as there is a predictable diurnal variation in blood levels. The lowest level is usually around midnight. Exercise increases cortisol levels. Because of the diurnal variation, multiple tests of cortisol levels are often conducted (such as at 8 a.m. and 4 p.m.) in order to evaluate the changes in levels. The total cortisol level—which is obtained with a 24-hour urine sample—does not show this variation. If there are abnormal findings, additional testing, such as dexamethasone suppression and ACTH stimulation, is often done.

78. A: If a patient sitting in a chair has a generalized convulsive seizure during venipuncture, the appropriate response is to discontinue venipuncture and call for help to ease the patient to the floor in order to avoid patient injury. The patient should be placed on one side if possible, but movements should not be restrained, and nothing should be placed in the patient's mouth. If possible, a pillow or blanket should be placed under the patient's head and restrictive clothing should be loosened. The time that the seizure begins and ends should be noted and first-aid personnel should be notified.

79. A: Alcohol, corticosteroids, blood pressure medications, and birth control pills may affect the results of a glucose tolerance test (GTT). Aspirin does not affect GTT results.

80. D: The nerve most often injured with venipuncture is the median nerve. Blood draws are most frequently done in the antecubital space, and the median nerve, which is the largest in the arm, passes through this area. The second most common injury is of the radial nerve, which runs near the cephalic vein on the radial side of the wrist and into the palm of the hand. Venipuncture should be avoided in the 7.5 cm area above the thumb.

81. D: When doing a venipuncture on a patient under investigation (PUI) for Ebola or with confirmed Ebola, the phlebotomist must use a combination of standard, contact, and droplet isolation plus enhanced measures because of the high risk of becoming infected with any contact with the patient's body fluids, including perspiration and droplets transmitted through coughing. The phlebotomist must follow Ebola protocols exactly, donning and removing PPE under direct supervision to ensure each step is carried out correctly.

82. D: If a sample is designated as QNS, the quantity is not sufficient for the test that has been ordered. In this case, the sample is rejected and another sample must be obtained. QNS is a common reason for rejecting chemistry specimens. The phlebotomist should review requirements for tests to ensure that the volume of the specimen is adequate. Reasons for QNS may include using expired tubes (resulting in decreased vacuum) and not ensuring complete filling of the tube before changing tubes. QNS may also occur if a patient has difficult-to-access veins.

83. D: Black-capped collection tubes are used only for ESR (erythrocyte sedimentation rate). These tubes contain sodium citrate as an additive. The ESR measures the number of red blood cells that fall to the bottom of the collection tube within an hour. The more that fall, the higher the sedimentation rate. The ESR is a non-specific test that indicates that an inflammatory process is occurring. Proteins that are produced in response to infection, cancer, or some autoimmune diseases promote clumping of the red blood cells, increasing the rate at which they fall.

84. B: Because microcollection tubes are used to collect very small volumes of capillary blood, such as from a fingerstick, they typically hold up to 0.5 mL of blood. These small containers, also sometimes referred to as "bullets" because of their miniature size, contain the same types of additives as larger evacuated tubes and the caps are color-coded in the same manner so that the additives can be easily identified.

85. C: When conducting the urine dipstick test, the dipstick should be dipped into the urine and then withdrawn and tapped lightly on the side of the container to remove excess urine. Then, the dipstick should be held in a horizontal position so that the urine on the dipstick pools and stays in contact with the reagents for the specified time period, usually ranging from 30 seconds to 2 minutes depending on the type of dipstick. Then, the dipstick is compared with a color chart to determine the results.

86. D: An appropriate question to verify a patient's ID is "Can you tell me your name and birthdate?" Asking for direct information is important because if a patient is confused or hard of hearing, he or she may answer "yes" or "no" to questions incorrectly. For inpatients, the ID band should always be checked to verify the information that they provide. If patients do not have an ID band, which is common in the outpatient setting, they should be asked to provide and spell their names and provide their birthdates.

87. C: If less than the recommended volume necessary for blood cultures is obtained, the aerobic specimen tube should be filled completely first and then the remainder is placed in the anaerobic tube. The tubes should be inverted gently a few times to prevent clotting. The only anticoagulant that is acceptable for blood cultures is sodium polyanetholesulfonate (SPS), and the blood can be collected directly into tubes with SPS and then transferred to the medium for culture.

88. C: A patient that falls and experiences a fractured hip will be treated in the orthopedic department, which specializes in caring for patients with impairments of or injuries to the skeletal system, including fractures. The oncology department specializes in the care of patients with cancer. Obstetrics specializes in the care of pregnant women, including labor and delivery. Outpatient departments, also commonly known as ambulatory care centers, provide same-day treatment and surgical procedures without hospital inpatient admission.

89. A: If a patient in the emergency department refuses to have blood drawn but the phlebotomist does so at the physician's insistence, the phlebotomist may be charged with assault. Unless the patient is a minor, legally deemed incompetent to make decisions, or is legally required to have a test (such as a blood alcohol level or tox-screen for illicit drugs), the individual has an absolute right to refuse any and all treatments and procedures.

90. C: If a phlebotomist develops dermatitis from all types of gloves, the best solution is to wear glove liners or apply a barrier hand cream specifically designed to prevent irritation from gloves.

Continuing to wear gloves, even for brief periods of time, may cause further irritation, which increases the risk of infection for both the phlebotomist and the patients. Additionally, if the hands are irritated, cleansing with alcohol-based rubs or soap and water may increase irritation.

91. D: Tests that can be run on cerebrospinal fluid (CSF) include total protein, glucose, and chloride. ABO typing is a blood test used to determine blood type; it may be used in paternity testing.

92. B: If a patient has severely impaired circulation in the legs and has had a recent bilateral mastectomy, the best choice for a blood draw is probably an artery. Blood cannot be drawn from the foot or ankle veins if the circulation is impaired, and blood should not be drawn from a vein on the side of a mastectomy, which (in this case) is bilateral, because the circulation may be impaired and edema may be present. An arterial blood draw is outside of the scope of practice of the phlebotomist.

93. B: All laboratory testing in the United States, except for research testing, is regulated by the Centers for Medicare & Medicaid Services (CMS) through the Clinical Laboratory Improvement Amendments (CLIA), which are implemented through the Division of Laboratory Services and serves approximately 244,000 laboratories. Laboratories receiving reimbursement from CMS must meet CLIA standards, which ensure that laboratory testing will be accurate and that procedures are followed properly.

94. C: Having multiple patients in one room introduces the most risk for error related to patient ID because the order may include the wrong bed assignment, so it is especially important to double-check the patient's ID. Because patients may be confused, the wristband should always be checked to verify the person's name. Other situations that increase the risk of error include tests on siblings (especially twins), newborns, people with common names (e.g., Mary Jones), and people with names that look alike or sound alike.

95. B: If an accidental arterial puncture is suspected, the correct response is to withdraw the needle immediately and apply strong pressure for a minimum of 5 minutes, observing the site carefully for signs of swelling or bleeding. The ordering physician must be notified, and an incident report must be completed. If a specimen was already collected before an arterial puncture was suspected, the laboratory may still be able to test the arterial blood.

96. A: Phlebotomists are especially at risk for developing an allergic response to latex because it is commonly used in tourniquets, gloves, and other medical equipment and devices, such as blood pressure cuffs. Contact dermatitis is frequently the first indication of an allergic response, but reactions can be severe, including anaphylaxis. Because some patients are also sensitive to latex, non-latex gloves and tourniquets should be used whenever possible.

97. B: The peak time for most drugs after intramuscular injection is approximately 60 minutes, whereas the peak time after IV administration is approximately 30 minutes. Oral medications, on the other hand, usually peak after 1-2 hours. Peak levels are assessed to ensure that the patient is not receiving a toxic dose of medication. Medications that are assessed with therapeutic drug monitoring typically have a narrow therapeutic range.

98. D: The thyroid-stimulating hormone (TSH) test is used to assess thyroid function; *GH* stands for "growth hormone," and *ADH* stands for "antidiuretic hormone." *GTT* is the abbreviation for "glucose tolerance test."

99. C: Warming of the injection site does not significantly affect the levels of routinely tested analytes. Warming is preferred for heelstick procedures in infants because warming increases blood flow. Warming is required for collection of blood gas or capillary pH specimens, and may be required before fingersticks in patients with cold hands.

100. D: The coronal (frontal) plane is parallel to the long axis of the body and divides the body into front (anterior) and back (posterior) sections. The sagittal plane divides the body into right and left sections; the midsagittal plane divides the body into equal right and left halves. The transverse plane divides the body into top and bottom sections.

101. D: The cortisol test requires a timed specimen. Because cortisol levels vary during the day, the blood for the test is usually drawn first thing in the morning. In some cases, patients are administered 1 mg of dexamethasone the night before the test. Patients are typically asked to avoid strenuous exercise for 24 hours before the test, and some medications that can affect the test results, including anticonvulsants, estrogens, synthetic steroids, and androgens, may be held.

102. C: If a phlebotomist obtains a blood sample and then accidentally experiences a needlestick that does not draw blood, the phlebotomist should wash the site with soap and water. The incident must be reported as soon as possible to a supervisor, and needlestick protocol should be followed. This may include testing and/or prophylaxis for communicable diseases such as HIV, depending on the patient's health history. In some cases, the patient may also be tested for communicable diseases in order to determine the risk to the phlebotomist.

103. B: When collecting a specimen from a patient in a long-term-care facility, the first thing that the phlebotomist should do is to check in at the nursing station. The phlebotomist needs to ask for information about any special concerns regarding the patient, such as the need for assistance if the patient is confused or any type of restriction that applies to the patient. As in any other setting, the phlebotomist should always knock on the door or announce his or her arrival before entering the room and explain the purpose of the visit.

104. A: If a specimen must be chilled, the best method is to place the specimen in a water-and-ice mixture so that adequate contact is made. Placing it in or on ice alone is not adequate because the cold will not be applied uniformly. Refrigerating the specimen cools it too slowly, and placing it in dry ice poses the risk that hemolysis may occur because of the extreme temperature change. Whole blood specimens are not usually chilled.

105. C: At room temperature, which is around 20–25 °C (68–77 °F), complete clotting usually occurs within 30–60 minutes. Chilling the specimen will delay the clotting time, and the clotting time will be prolonged in patients who are receiving anticoagulants. Some collection devices contain activators to speed up the clotting time if the sample must be tested quickly. For example, thrombin results in coagulation within 5 minutes, and glass/silica particles result in coagulation within 15–30 minutes.

106. D: Cerebrospinal fluid (CSF) is usually collected in three or four numbered tubes. If four tubes are collected, they are tested in the following manner:

1. Chemistry and immunology tests
2. Microbiology studies
3. Cell count and differential
4. Cytology and special tests

The cell count is conducted with the third tube that is collected because the first two tubes are more likely to be contaminated with blood cells that were introduced during the spinal tap.

107. C: The throat is also known as the pharynx. The larynx is known as the voice box. The trachea is known as the windpipe. The epiglottis is a covering of the opening of the larynx that causes food to pass down the esophagus rather than the trachea.

108. D: The most common reason for rejecting a specimen for chemistry is hemolysis, whereas the most common reason for rejecting a specimen for hematology is clotting. Other reasons that specimens may be rejected include overfilling or underfilling a tube, because this alters the required ratio of additive to specimen and can interfere with the testing results. Specimens transported and handled in the wrong collection tube, at the wrong temperature, with the wrong additive, or with exposure to light (if photosensitive) may also be rejected.

109. B: CLSI guidelines recommend for pediatric patients that the amount of blood drawn in 24 hours be no more than 5% of the patient's total blood volume. Using 75 mL/kg as the estimate for blood volume, calculate the child's total blood volume:

$$29 \text{ lb} \times \frac{1 \text{ kg}}{2.2 \text{ lb}} = 13.2 \text{ kg}$$

$$13.2 \text{ kg} \times 75 \frac{\text{mL}}{\text{kg}} = 990 \text{ mL}$$

The maximum volume of blood that can be drawn from this patient in 24 hours is 5% of that total volume, which is approximately 50 mL. Care must be taken to avoid withdrawing more than 5% of the child's total blood volume in a 24-hr period. Additionally, the phlebotomist must consider the maximum blood volume that can be withdrawn within longer time periods. CLSI regulations limit the amount of blood drawn over an 8-week period to no more than 10% of the patient's total blood volume.

110. D: Strenuous exercise may increase values of lactic dehydrogenase (LD) and creatinine phosphokinase (CPK) for more than 24 hours after exercise stops. Even mild exercise may increase some laboratory values for a short period of time, but these changes dissipate so quickly that they rarely affect findings. Short-term changes in lactic acid, protein, creatinine, and some enzymes may occur after exercise. The degree to which exercise affects laboratory values depends on the type of exercise and the amount of time between exercise and testing.

111. A: Plasma specimens for ammonia levels should be separated from the blood cells and tested within 15 minutes because ammonia levels increase rapidly at room temperature. Specimens should be transported in an ice slurry or cooling tray and processed immediately. Blood ammonia levels are often checked to diagnose or monitor hepatic encephalopathy, which can result in toxic levels of ammonia. Other causes of increased ammonia include upper gastrointestinal tract bleeding, salicylate poisoning, liver failure, kidney disease, and parenteral nutrition.

112. D: Control runs of automated systems should be carried out at the beginning of each day to ensure that the equipment is fully operational. Automated systems carry out laboratory tests with little input from personnel once the equipment is loaded with the appropriate samples. Automated systems may produce errors; therefore, close monitoring is essential. Routine maintenance should be carried out on a scheduled basis. Maintenance may include cleaning spills, changing reagents, discarding waste, changing parts as needed, and making adjustments.

113. D: Serous fluid may be obtained from the peritoneal (abdominal) cavity, the pleural cavity surrounding the lungs, or the pericardial cavity surrounding the heart. Cerebrospinal fluid is obtained from the spinal cavity.

114. D: The additive that is most effective at preserving coagulation factors is sodium citrate. Light-blue–capped evacuated collection tubes contain sodium citrate and are used for coagulation tests, which are conducted on plasma. The volume ratio of blood to anticoagulant must be 9:1 to obtain the correct clotting times, so the tubes must be filled to capacity, and both overfilling and underfilling must be avoided. The collection tubes must be inverted immediately to prevent activation of clotting, but shaking or mixing vigorously must be avoided because it may activate platelets and decrease clotting times.

115. A: When collecting a blood specimen from a patient in an isolation room, the phlebotomist should collect the needed supplies and place the collection tray at the nurse's station or in another secured area. The tray should not be left unattended in a public area. Any supplies taken into the isolation room are considered contaminated and cannot then be used for other patients, so they must be properly disposed of. Tourniquets used for isolation rooms should be dedicated to the patient or disposable.

116. A: If a patient had a right mastectomy 6 months previously, blood may be drawn from the left arm. Blood generally should not be obtained on the side of a mastectomy, regardless of the length of time since surgery. Any degree of lymphedema may alter the results of the blood tests, and the patient is at increased risk of infection from venipuncture. If no other site is available, a physician's order should be obtained regarding use of this site before attempting to withdraw blood from the side of the mastectomy.

117. C: Safety features for venipuncture needles may not be detachable but rather must be a permanent integral part of the needle. The safety feature must ensure that the hands stay behind the needle and must be activated by one hand only. The safety feature should be easy to use and remain in place when the needle is discarded. Safety features may sheathe, blunt, or retract the needle after use, depending on the manufacturer.

118. A: If a blood specimen is to be obtained for the trough (lowest blood concentration) level of a drug, the best time to draw the blood is usually 15 minutes before the next scheduled dose because the concentration should be at its lowest point. Trough levels may be checked to ensure that a minimum amount of drug remains in the blood. The levels may also be used to determine the correct dose and spacing of doses and to help determine the rate of drug absorption.

119. A: The infections most commonly transmitted through needlestick and sharp injuries are HBV (hepatitis B virus), HCV (hepatitis C virus), and HIV (human immunodeficiency virus). While these viruses pose the greatest risk—and people may be co-infected, putting the person who has a needlestick or sharp injury at risk of more than one disease—more than 20 other infectious disorders can also be spread through needlesticks and sharps injuries. These include syphilis, HZV (herpes zoster virus), toxoplasmosis, TB (tuberculosis), Rocky Mountain spotted fever, blastomycosis, and cutaneous gonorrhea.

120. D: The specimen for a lactic acid test must be chilled. Other tests that require a chilled specimen include catecholamines, ammonia, pyruvate, adrenocorticotropic hormone, parathyroid hormone, metanephrines (plasma), and gastrin. Chilling the specimen slows the cell metabolism that otherwise continues and protects analytes that are altered by heat. Most specimens that require chilling are chilled in an ice-and-water slurry. A few specimens, such as homocysteine in the gel tube, are chilled on a cooler rack.

Practice Test #2

1. Which of the following are patients NOT prohibited from ingesting prior to a fecal occult blood test?

    a. Vitamin C
    b. Aspirin
    c. Spinach
    d. Horseradish

2. If an elderly patient has rolling veins, which of the following is the best solution?

    a. Apply a tourniquet immediately above the venipuncture site.
    b. Use a winged infusion set with a syringe.
    c. Use a winged infusion set with evacuated tubes.
    d. Anchor the vein with the thumb.

3. When conducting a fingerstick glucose test, to transfer the blood from the finger to the test strip, the phlebotomist should:

    a. Hold the edge of the strip next to the drop of blood.
    b. Dip the strip directly into the drop of blood.
    c. Wipe the strip across the drop of blood.
    d. Use a disposable pipette for transfer.

4. All of the following are indicative of a UTI EXCEPT:

    a. Leukocytes
    b. Nitrites
    c. Protein
    d. Glucose

5. For therapeutic drug monitoring, critical times include:

    a. The time of the last dose and the time the specimen was collected
    b. The time of the last dose and the time the specimen was examined
    c. The time the specimen was collected and the time the specimen was examined
    d. The time the specimen was collected

6. Which of the following tubes can be used for testing ethanol level?

    a. Light-blue–capped
    b. Royal-blue–capped
    c. Gray-capped
    d. Green-capped

7. Underfilling a green-capped evacuated collection tube may result in:

    a. Low test results
    b. Clotting
    c. Cell morphology changes
    d. No adverse effects

8. When delivering a blood specimen that requires STAT testing to the laboratory, the phlebotomist must:

    a. Ensure that the specimen is marked as STAT.
    b. Place it in a STAT rack.
    c. Assume that the testing personnel are aware of the STAT request.
    d. Notify the testing personnel of the STAT request and receive verbal acknowledgement.

9. Which of the following statements regarding arterial puncture is FALSE?

    a. The patient should be checked for allergies before the procedure.
    b. A patient afraid of needles should be calmed down.
    c. A phlebotomist may be trained to perform the procedure.
    d. The chance of a hematoma is increased.

10. If the phlebotomist is accidently splashed with a highly toxic hazardous chemical, what is the minimum length of time that the affected body part should be flushed with water?

    a. 2 minutes
    b. 5 minutes
    c. 10 minutes
    d. 15 minutes

11. A person with blood type AB+ should receive a transfusion of blood type:

    a. A+
    b. B+
    c. AB+
    d. A+, B+, or AB+

12. The hydrogen breath test is most often used to test for:

    a. *H. pylori* infection
    b. Irritable bowel syndrome
    c. Small-intestine bacterial overgrowth
    d. Lactose intolerance

13. The ratio of blood to additive in evacuated collection tubes that contain sodium citrate or ACD must be:

    a. 10 : 1
    b. 9 : 1
    c. 8 : 2
    d. 7 : 3

14. Which of the following governmental agencies requires an exposure control plan that outlines methods to reduce staff injury and exposure?

    a. CMS
    b. OSHA
    c. TJC
    d. CDC

15. If a phlebotomist is asked to transport a nonblood specimen, such as a urine sample, to the laboratory for testing, the phlebotomist should:
- a. Accept the specimen for transport.
- b. Verify that the sample is labeled correctly.
- c. Refuse to accept the specimen for transport.
- d. Check with the laboratory supervisor regarding the transport.

16. In therapeutic drug monitoring, sample collection timing is MOST critical for:
- a. Phenobarbital
- b. Digoxin
- c. Ethanol
- d. Aminoglycosides

17. If a patient's test request requires a chemistry panel, a CBC, a PT, and blood typing, in what order should the specimens be drawn, first to last?
- a. CBC, chemistry panel, PT, blood typing
- b. Chemistry panel, PT, blood typing, CBC
- c. PT, blood typing, CBC, chemistry panel
- d. PT, chemistry panel, blood typing, and CBC

18. If protocol for blood C&S requires skin antisepsis with alcohol (70% isopropyl) followed by tincture of iodine (2%), but the patient is allergic to iodine, an acceptable alternate procedure is:
- a. Wash with soap and water and cleanse once with alcohol.
- b. Cleanse twice with alcohol.
- c. Cleanse 3 times with alcohol.
- d. Wash with soap and water and cleanse twice with alcohol.

19. Which of the following actions by a phlebotomist should NOT result in a lawsuit for negligence?
- a. Doing a fingerstick on a 6-month-old infant
- b. Providing information about a test to a child's mother
- c. Misidentifying a patient
- d. Lowering a bed rail and leaving it down

20. Which government agency is responsible for regulations governing the use of gloves when carrying out a venipuncture?
- a. USDA
- b. FDA
- c. CDC
- d. OSHA

21. Which of the following is a method of preventing reflux of a collection-tube additive?
- a. Allow back and forth movement in the tube while filling.
- b. Maintain the arm in a downward position while filling the tube.
- c. Maintain the arm in an upward position while filling the tube.
- d. Hold the collection tube very still while filling.

22. Which of the following should NOT be disposed of in a sharps container?

a. Bloodstained gauze
b. Tube holder
c. Lancet
d. Opened but clean needle

23. Abnormal bone development caused by a lack of vitamin D in the diet is known as:

a. Arthritis
b. Osteochondritis
c. Rickets
d. Osteomyelitis

24. Which of the following steps can help prevent the development of a hematoma?

a. Maintain the position of the needle throughout the specimen collection.
b. Remove the needle before removing the tourniquet.
c. Remove the needle before removing the tube from the holder.
d. Bandage the puncture site immediately after needle removal.

25. Which of the following may violate the chain of custody for a forensic specimen?

a. Signing the chain of custody form
b. Asking a nurse to temporarily store the specimen
c. Placing the specimen in a transfer bag
d. Documenting the patient's identification

26. Which of the following is a health hazard as opposed to a physical hazard?

a. Compressed gas
b. Combustible liquid
c. Explosive material
d. Corrosive chemical

27. For pediatric or critically ill patients, what percentage of total blood volume can be collected within a 24-hour period?

a. <1%
b. 1–5%
c. 6–8%
d. 10%

28. If petechiae are noted on the patient's skin distal to the tourniquet, this suggests that:

a. The tourniquet has been improperly applied.
b. The patient is having an allergic reaction.
c. The patient may have a coagulation defect.
d. The tourniquet has been on for too long.

29. HCV exposure may occur through:

a. Urine
b. Sexual contact
c. Semen
d. Phlebotomy procedures

30. During venipuncture, if the needle appears to be in the vein but no blood is flowing and a slight vibration or quiver of the needle is noted, the most appropriate initial response is to:

   a. Immediately discontinue the venipuncture.

   b. Remove the vacuum tube, pull back slightly on the needle, and reinsert the vacuum tube.

   c. Rotate the needle slightly to the right or left.

   d. Remove the vacuum tube, gently insert the needle further, and reinsert the vacuum tube.

31. If a venipuncture is requested at a specific time but the phlebotomist mistakenly collects the specimen 30 minutes late, the phlebotomist should:

   a. Report the late collection immediately.

   b. Assume that 30 minutes is within an acceptable range of time.

   c. Write the time of collection on the label.

   d. Do or say nothing about the late collection unless asked.

32. For which of the following tests must the blood specimen be maintained at body temperature until processing?

   a. Cold agglutinins

   b. Lactic acid

   c. PH

   d. Parathyroid hormone

33. If the phlebotomist notes that a previous venipuncture site is tender and erythematous with a red streak extending 4 inches above the site, the likely cause is:

   a. Allergic response

   b. Hematoma

   c. Ecchymosis

   d. Phlebitis

34. What is the purpose of a Vein Entry Indicator Device (VEID)?

   a. Indicate when a needle penetrates a vein.

   b. Identify the pattern of veins.

   c. Differentiate arteries from veins.

   d. Prevent hematomas from venipuncture.

35. Serum that appears milky likely indicates:

   a. Lipemia

   b. Bacterial infection

   c. Viral infection

   d. Dehydration

36. In double-pointed needles, the rubber sheath that covers the shorter needle is intended to:

   a. Prevent needlestick injuries.

   b. Prevent leakage of blood.

   c. Indicate the side used for venipuncture.

   d. Prevent breakage of the needle.

37. Alcohol-based antisepsis is more commonly used than povidone-iodine–based antisepsis because:

    a. Alcohol is more effective.
    b. Alcohol is less expensive.
    c. Povidone-iodine is more irritating to the skin.
    d. Povidone-iodine is more likely to cause an allergic response.

38. What is the cap color of the collection tube for PT, aPTT, and TT?

    a. Green
    b. Lavender
    c. Light blue
    d. Gray

39. The primary purpose of therapeutic drug monitoring (TDM) is to:

    a. Identify optimal dosing.
    b. Determine abuse of drugs.
    c. Wean patient off of drugs.
    d. Prevent adverse effects.

40. If a patient is very thin and has prominent veins that require a low needle angle for venipuncture, the best choice is probably:

    a. 21-gauge needle with tube holder
    b. Winged infusion set with syringe
    c. 21-gauge needle with syringe
    d. 23-gauge needle with syringe

41. Venipuncture of which of the following veins poses the greatest risk of accidental puncture of an artery?

    a. Median cubital vein
    b. Cephalic
    c. Basilic vein
    d. Metacarpal vein

42. A patient lying on their stomach is said to be in the:

    a. Anatomic position
    b. Prone position
    c. Supine position
    d. Reclining position

43. After a needle and tube holder are used to collect a blood specimen, the tube holder should be:

    a. Separated from the needle for reuse
    b. Separated from the needle for disposal in the hazardous waste container
    c. Disposed of as one unit with the needle in the sharps container
    d. Separated from the needle and disposed of in an open waste container

44. When asked to collect blood from a peripheral vascular access device, the phlebotomist should recognize that this procedure:

 a. Is outside his or her scope of practice
 b. Requires supervision
 c. Requires additional training
 d. Is contraindicated

45. When loading a centrifuge that holds multiple tubes, if only one tube needs to be centrifuged, the phlebotomist should:

 a. Place the single tube in the centrifuge and complete the centrifugation.
 b. Place the tube and an empty tube across from it in the centrifuge.
 c. Place the tube and a tube filled with the same volume of water across from it in the centrifuge.
 d. Wait until another blood sample is available and then centrifuge both.

46. If blood cannot be obtained from either arm, before using a foot or ankle for drawing blood, the phlebotomist must:

 a. Check with a supervisor.
 b. Obtain a physician's order.
 c. Ask the patient's permission.
 d. Review the procedure.

47. The normal range for blood glucose level in a healthy adult is:

 a. 65–110 mg/dL
 b. 45–65 mg/dL
 c. 55–75 mg/dL
 d. 45–90 mg/dL

48. When carrying out POC testing for PT/INR with an analyzer such as the CoaguChek XS Plus, a capillary blood drop should generally be applied to the test strip or other collection device within:

 a. 5 seconds
 b. 10 seconds
 c. 15 seconds
 d. 20 seconds

49. Which of the following items requires disinfection?

 a. Surgical instruments
 b. Blood pressure cuffs
 c. Furniture in the waiting area
 d. Windows

50. OSHA requires that a HEPA respirator be used for:

 a. Enteric isolation
 b. Caring for burn patients
 c. Contact isolation
 d. Caring for AFB patients

51. When using an evacuated tube system for venipuncture, how can the phlebotomist determine that the needle is correctly positioned in the vein?

  a. A flash of blood is seen at the hub.
  b. Blood flows into the holder.
  c. The needle slightly vibrates.
  d. The phlebotomist feels a decrease in resistance.

52. In an inpatient facility, PPE for the phlebotomist must be provided by:

  a. The phlebotomist
  b. The employer
  c. The FDA
  d. OSHA

53. If a laboratory detects a suspected outbreak of an infectious disease, such as *E. coli* infections, to which governmental agency should a report be made?

  a. CLSI
  b. CDC
  c. NIH
  d. Local or state health department

54. Before a blood specimen is collected from a newborn for routine screening for inborn errors of metabolism (IEM), the infant should:

  a. Have been nursed or bottle-fed for at least 12 hours
  b. Have been nursed or bottle-fed for at least 24 hours
  c. Have not been nursed or bottle-fed for at least 2 hours
  d. Have not been nursed or bottle-fed for at least 4 hours

55. The primary use of non-additive evacuated plastic collection tubes is for:

  a. Practice tubes
  b. Cultures
  c. Contaminated samples
  d. Discard tubes

56. Which of the following supplies is NOT needed for routine venipuncture?

  a. Cotton balls
  b. Gauze sponges
  c. Tube holders
  d. Needles

57. If blood must be drawn from an arm with an IV in place, the phlebotomist should:

  a. Turn off the IV and wait at least 2 minutes before attempting venipuncture.
  b. Ask the nurse to turn off the IV and wait 2 minutes before attempting venipuncture.
  c. Place a tourniquet proximal to the IV and carry out venipuncture distal to the IV.
  d. Place a tourniquet proximal to the IV and carry out venipuncture proximal to the IV.

58. **Which of the following evacuated collection tubes should NOT be used to collect a specimen for a BMP?**

a. Red-capped with clot activator
b. Red/Black -capped SST
c. Lavender-capped
d. Green-capped

59. **An electrolyte panel includes:**

a. HCO_3, Cl, K, and Na
b. CO_2, Cl, Ca, and K
c. Cl, K, Na, and CO_2
d. CO_2, PO_4, Na, and K

60. **Physician office laboratories are most often accredited by:**

a. CLIA
b. COLA
c. CAP
d. The Joint Commission

61. **For venipuncture, the vein should be anchored:**

a. On the right or left of the puncture site (one finger)
b. On the right and left of the puncture site (two fingers)
c. Proximal to the puncture site
d. Distal to the puncture site

62. **Which of the following tests should be available on a POC ABG analyzer?**

a. PCO_2
b. Hgb
c. Na
d. Hct

63. **When carrying out a heelstick blood collection on a newborn, what should the maximum depth of the puncture be?**

a. 1 mm
b. 1.5 mm
c. 2 mm
d. 3 mm

64. **Which stopper color indicates the correct tube for a CBC?**

a. Lavender/purple
b. Light blue
c. Pink
d. Green

65. **For venipuncture, which vein should always be selected as the last option?**

a. Median cubital
b. Cephalic
c. Basilic
d. Dorsal metacarpal

66. In which order should green capped, lavender-capped, and red-capped pediatric micro-collection containers be collected?

    a. Green, lavender, and red

    b. Lavender, green, and red

    c. Red, lavender, and green

    d. Lavender, red, and green

67. In administering a TB test:

    a. The antigen must be injected into a vein.

    b. The antigen must be injected just below the skin.

    c. The degree of erythema is measured to determine a reaction.

    d. Presence of a bleb, or wheal, indicates the antigen was injected improperly.

68. If a gray-capped collection tube is overfilled, the result may be:

    a. No effect

    b. Low test result

    c. High test result

    d. Clotting of the specimen

69. Which of the following agencies provides standards for performance and testing of all types of laboratory functions, including clinical microbiology?

    a. CLSI

    b. WHO

    c. NCQA

    d. CLIAC

70. If a venipuncture is required from an elderly patient with obvious tremors of the upper extremities, the best solution is to:

    a. Ask the patient to keep the arm still.

    b. Ask a nurse to assist in stabilizing the arm.

    c. Use an ankle or foot vein.

    d. Refuse to do the venipuncture.

71. Which of the following vein-finder devices projects a pattern map of the veins on the skin?

    a. Ultrasound

    b. Near-infrared light

    c. Transilluminator

    d. Vein-finder glasses

72. Sputum specimens should ideally be obtained:

    a. After 4 hours of fasting

    b. First thing in the morning upon arising

    c. At any time of day

    d. In the evening just before bed

73. If a very small hematoma is evident during venipuncture, the best initial response is to:
   a. Remove the needle, elevate the arm, and apply pressure.
   b. Remove the needle and apply an ice compress.
   c. Remove the needle and apply pressure.
   d. Observe and complete the venipuncture.

74. The greatest risk when a tube breaks during centrifugation is:
   a. Aerosolization of sample
   b. Lacerations/Puncture wounds
   c. Equipment damage
   d. Electric shock

75. For forensic collection of a blood sample, the specimen container must be:
   a. Placed and sealed inside a transfer bag
   b. Taped shut
   c. Personally observed during testing
   d. Placed in a clear plastic bag

76. According to the ADA, to ensure accessibility to patients on crutches or in wheelchairs, at least one space next to the phlebotomy chair must have a minimum area of:
   a. 20 × 30 inches
   b. 30 × 48 inches
   c. 36 × 60 inches
   d. 48 × 72 inches

77. When the phlebotomist is using microcollection tubes for a fingerstick, the collection tube that should usually be filled first is:
   a. Gray-capped
   b. Lavender-capped
   c. Green-capped
   d. Yellow-capped

78. When collecting a capillary blood specimen for bilirubin from a newborn receiving phototherapy for jaundice, it is especially important to:
   a. Work as quickly as possible.
   b. Collect the specimen in a clear container.
   c. Turn off the phototherapy light during collection.
   d. Avoid blocking the phototherapy lights.

79. The correct method of removing a stopper from a specimen tube is to:
   a. Twist the stopper off.
   b. Pull it straight up and away from the tube.
   c. Pop the stopper off by applying pressure on one side with a thumb.
   d. Use forceps to grasp the stopper and pull it from the tube.

80. Which of the following billing code systems is used for laboratory testing for inpatients?

   a. ICD-11
   b. ICD-10-PCS
   c. ICD-10-CM
   d. CPT

81. If the phlebotomist drops an unused glass collection tube, causing it to break and scatter pieces of glass, the phlebotomist should:

   a. Clean up the glass with a wet paper towel.
   b. Ask the nursing staff to clean up the glass.
   c. Guard the area and notify housekeeping.
   d. Notify a supervisor.

82. For blood cultures, if using iodophors for the main disinfectant, how long does it take for the iodophors to adequately disinfect the skin?

   a. 15–30 seconds
   b. 30–60 seconds
   c. 60–90 seconds
   d. 90–120 seconds

83. Metal filings ("fleas") may be used with capillary blood glass collection tubes to:

   a. Seal the tube ends.
   b. Collect the blood sample.
   c. Conduct the heelstick.
   d. Mix blood with anticoagulant.

84. Which of the following tests is typically ordered STAT?

   a. pCO_2
   b. HCG
   c. FBS
   d. Hgb

85. The Joint Commission is primarily a(n):

   a. Research facility
   b. Regulatory agency
   c. FDA advisory board
   d. Accrediting organization

86. The phlebotomist should evaluate the risk of violence with:

   a. Confused patients
   b. All patients
   c. Inebriated patients
   d. Angry patients

87. When opening and aliquoting a specimen, the required PPE includes:

   a. Gloves
   b. Gown and gloves
   c. Gown, gloves, N95 respirator, and face shield
   d. Gown, gloves, and face shield

88. Blood draws for a GTT in pregnancy are usually done at _____ after the test begins.

   a. 30 minutes, 1 hour, 2 hours, and 4 hours
   b. 30 minutes, 60 minutes, 90 minutes, and 2 hours
   c. 2 hours, 4 hours, 6 hours, and 8 hours
   d. 1 hour, 2 hours, and 3 hours

89. When using a pediatric vein transilluminator with an infant, the transilluminator should be:

   a. Placed in the palm of the child's hand
   b. Held in place over the veins by a second person
   c. Placed in a holder above the puncture site
   d. Run along the surface of the skin to illuminate the veins

90. For which of the following tests must blood be drawn from an artery?

   a. Anti-hemophilic factor
   b. Chromosome analysis
   c. Hemoglobin A1c
   d. Blood gases

91. The first step in carrying out a venipuncture is to:

   a. Explain the purpose.
   b. Obtain consent.
   c. Identify the patient.
   d. Identify the site.

92. Which of the following is NOT commonly associated with nosocomial infections?

   a. *Klebsiella pneumoniae*
   b. *Mycobacterium tuberculosis*
   c. MRSA
   d. *Clostridioides difficile*

93. In the United States, all laboratory testing, except for research, is regulated by:

   a. CMS
   b. FDA
   c. CAP
   d. OSHA

94. If the phlebotomist observes another worker placing needles and syringes into a personal bag before leaving work, the best response is to:

   a. Confront the worker.
   b. Remain quiet.
   c. Call the police.
   d. Notify a supervisor.

95. Which of the following tests is used to identify the medications that can be prescribed to treat a UTI?

   a. ACTH
   b. TSH
   c. C&S
   d. FBS

96. All of the following affect blood specimen composition EXCEPT:

   a. Body position
   b. Temperature and humidity
   c. Fasting
   d. Stress

97. Separated serum or plasma specimens should be maintained at room temperature for no more than:

   a. 2 hours
   b. 4 hours
   c. 6 hours
   d. 8 hours

98. If an indwelling line, such as a central venous catheter, is used to obtain a blood sample, how much blood should be discarded before the sample is collected?

   a. 1 mL
   b. 2 mL
   c. 4 mL
   d. 5 mL

99. Which of the following is NOT normally present in urine?

   a. Ketones
   b. Bilirubin
   c. Albumin
   d. Bacteria

100. If the phlebotomist is asked to draw blood from a hospitalized patient who has lost her armband, the first action the phlebotomist should take is to:

   a. Ask staff to replace the armband.
   b. Ask the patient for two identifiers.
   c. Verify the patient's identification with staff.
   d. Verify the correct room number.

101. A test request should include what specific information about the patient?

   a. Name, identification (ID)/record number, gender, and date of birth
   b. Name, date of birth, and address
   c. Gender, ID/record number, indication for the test, and date of birth
   d. Name, ID/record number, telephone number, and date of birth

102. If a patient is very angry and yells that the lab tests are a "waste of time," which of the following is the best initial response?
a. Stay calm and listen.
b. Explain the purpose of the tests.
c. Leave the room.
d. Ask the patient to be civil.

103. If a patient has paralysis and lack of sensation in the right arm and hand, the best choice for venipuncture is:
a. Any appropriate site on the right arm
b. The dorsal metacarpal veins on the right hand
c. Any appropriate site on the right or left arm
d. Any appropriate site on the left arm

104. When transporting a specimen at room temperature, an appropriate temperature is:
a. 37 °C
b. 34 °C
c. 22 °C
d. 18 °C

105. If a patient is chewing gum when the phlebotomist arrives to collect a blood specimen, the phlebotomist should:
a. Ask the patient to stop chewing during the venipuncture.
b. Ask the patient to remove the gum before proceeding.
c. Tell the patient to be careful not to swallow the gum.
d. Ignore the fact that the patient is chewing gum.

106. When using an evacuated tube system for venipuncture, the phlebotomist can determine that a tube is properly filled when the:
a. Vacuum is exhausted.
b. Volume fills to the "full" line.
c. Volume fills the tube completely.
d. Volume appears adequate on examination.

107. If a phlebotomist sustains a needlestick injury, the first step is to:
a. Notify the supervisor.
b. Cleanse the puncture site with alcohol-based hand rub.
c. Wash the puncture site with soap and water.
d. Milk the wound to promote bleeding.

108. Using a foot vein for a blood draw:
a. Is prohibited
b. Poses no increased risks
c. Increases risk of blood clots
d. Is negligent

109. When drawing a blood specimen from an adolescent, the phlebotomist should recognize that most adolescents are:

    a. Self-conscious
    b. Belligerent
    c. Fearful
    d. Disinterested

110. The preferred capillary puncture site for adults and children older than 1 year of age is the:

    a. Lateral heel
    b. Distal segment of the nondominant third or fourth finger
    c. Distal segment of the dominant third or fourth finger
    d. Earlobe

111. The chain of custody for a blood specimen begins with the:

    a. Order
    b. Initial patient contact
    c. Transfer to the lab
    d. Processing

112. The order of draw is determined by the:

    a. FDA
    b. CAP
    c. JCAHO
    d. CLSI

113. The abbreviation for the thyroid hormone triiodothyronine is:

    a. T3
    b. T4
    c. TSH
    d. TBG

114. Which of the following is NOT a reason to avoid removing stoppers from blood specimen tubes prior in the precentrifugation period?

    a. To prevent a decrease in pH
    b. To prevent a loss of CO_2
    c. To prevent concentration of the specimen
    d. To prevent contamination

115. Which of the following statements regarding blood specimens is FALSE?

    a. Outpatient and inpatient blood specimens have the same normal values.
    b. Hemoglobin and hematocrit have higher normal ranges at higher elevations.
    c. Caffeine may affect cortisol levels.
    d. Ingestion of butter or cheese may produce a milky specimen.

116. A blood sample in a gray-capped evacuated collection tube should be inverted a minimum of:

    a. 5 times

    b. 6 times

    c. 8 times

    d. 12 times

117. The closure cap of the collection tube that contains sodium citrate is:

    a. Gray

    b. Lavender

    c. Green

    d. Light blue

118. If a coagulation test requires platelet-poor plasma, it is necessary to:

    a. Centrifuge the specimen, remove three-quarters of the plasma into an aliquot tube, and centrifuge the aliquot.

    b. Centrifuge the specimen, let the specimen sit for 10 minutes, and centrifuge again.

    c. Centrifuge the specimen at twice the usual duration of time before removing the plasma.

    d. Centrifuge the specimen, remove half of the plasma into an aliquot tube, and centrifuge the specimen again.

119. Which of the following tests CANNOT be carried out on a specimen obtained through heelstick or other capillary blood sample?

    a. CBC

    b. Glucose (bedside)

    c. Blood gas analysis

    d. Blood cultures

120. How long after a patient undergoing a C-urea breath test has completed the baseline exhalation sample and swallowed the synthetic urea solution should the second exhalation sample be taken?

    a. 5 minutes

    b. 10 minutes

    c. 15 minutes

    d. 30 minutes

Answer Key and Explanations for Test #2

1. C: Prior to a fecal occult blood test, patients are prohibited from ingesting certain foods (e.g., red meat, turnips, and horseradish), supplements (e.g., vitamin C), and medications (e.g., aspirin and anti-inflammatory drugs). However, patients are encouraged to eat fruits such as prunes, grapes, and apples and vegetables such as spinach, lettuce, and corn.

2. D: If an elderly patient has rolling veins, the best solution is to anchor the vein with the thumb directly distal to the puncture site, applying slight downward pressure to stretch and hold the vein in place. Rolling veins are common in elderly adults of both genders because the supportive tissue is weaker and fails to secure the vein. The arm should be extended as much as possible if using the antecubital space for the venipuncture.

3. A: When conducting a fingerstick glucose test, to transfer the blood from the finger to the test strip, the phlebotomist should hold the edge of the strip next to the drop of blood. The blood will wick onto the strip. For most tests, the first drop should be wiped away, and the second drop is used for testing. Before testing, controls should be run to ensure that the control solution and the control strips match. After the puncture site is cleansed with alcohol, the alcohol should be allowed to completely dry before proceeding.

4. D: A positive nitrite test in conjunction with a positive leukocyte test is indicative of urinary tract infection (UTI); a urine culture positive for blood or protein is also indicative of UTI. Glucose in the urine may be indicative of diabetes mellitus.

5. A: For therapeutic drug monitoring, critical times include the time of the last dose and the time that the specimen was collected. The times should be carefully recorded to ensure that the peak level or trough level is accurately assessed. Peak levels are drawn at the time that the medication's concentration in the blood should be highest. Trough levels are usually drawn immediately before the next dose, when the concentration is the lowest. The last dosage administered and the mode of administration must also be recorded.

6. C: The correct collection tube for testing ethanol (blood alcohol) level is the gray-capped tube that contains the antiglycolytic agent sodium fluoride. Antiglycolytics are agents that prevent glucose from breaking down, so the gray-capped collection tube is also used to check glucose levels (fasting blood sugar, or FBS). Because glycolysis can break down ethanol and decrease ethanol levels, the specimen for an ethanol test must be collected in a tube with an antiglycolytic.

7. A: Underfilling a green-capped evacuated collection tube may result in low test results because this results in excess heparin and a dilution effect. The minimal acceptable draw volume for a green-capped collection tube is 50%. Overfilling, on the other hand, may result in insufficient heparin to prevent clotting, so clots may form. If this occurs, the blood sample must be discarded and a new specimen obtained. The green-capped tube may contain either lithium heparin or sodium heparin, and is used for chemistry tests on plasma.

8. D: When delivering a blood specimen that requires STAT (immediate) testing to the laboratory, the phlebotomist must notify the testing personnel and receive verbal acknowledgement of a STAT specimen. Even if a STAT rack is available, simply placing the specimen in the rack is not sufficient because personnel who are busily engaged in testing may not notice that a specimen has been placed in the rack, resulting in delays in getting the test results.

9. C: Only physicians or specially trained emergency room personnel are qualified to perform arterial puncture; a phlebotomist is not trained to perform this procedure. Patients should be checked for allergies and must be in a steady state; thus, a patient who is afraid of needles must be calmed before the procedure. The risk of hematoma is increased with arterial puncture.

10. D: If the phlebotomist is accidently splashed with a highly toxic hazardous chemical, the minimum length of time that the affected body part should be flushed with water is 15 minutes. The phlebotomist should know the locations of safety showers and eye wash stations and should immediately follow procedures for decontamination. Once the phlebotomist completes the shower or flushing of the affected body part, they should immediately go to an appropriate health service, such as the emergency department, for evaluation.

11. C: A person with blood type AB+ should receive a transfusion with blood type AB+. While blood type AB+ is considered the "universal recipient" because the person can receive A+, B+, AB+, or O+ blood types in an emergency, other types of blood may still have antibodies (anti-A or anti-B) that may in some cases cause agglutination. If it is necessary to administer a type different than AB+, then it should be administered slowly (usually as packed cells) and the patient monitored closely.

12. D: The hydrogen breath test is most often used to test for lactose intolerance. Typically, exhaled breath contains very little hydrogen. However, if there is a problem with the digestion of lactose or other carbohydrates (such as fructose), bacteria in the colon ferment the carbohydrates, and this produces hydrogen. The hydrogen is absorbed into the systemic circulation and sent to the lungs, then it is exhaled. Higher than normal levels of hydrogen suggest a problem with carbohydrate metabolism.

13. B: The ratio of blood to additive in evacuated collection tubes that contain sodium citrate or ACD (acid citrate dextrose) must be 9:1 (draw to the 10 mL marking). Sodium citrate and ACD are both anticoagulants that stop blood from clotting in the collection tube. Maintaining the proper ratio is important to ensure that the anticoagulant has the correct effect. Sodium citrate is in light-blue–capped tubes and ACD is in yellow-capped tubes.

14. B: The governmental agency that requires an exposure control plan that outlines methods to reduce staff injury and exposure is the Occupational Safety and Health Administration (OSHA). OSHA requires that the working environment and working conditions be safe and free of recognized dangers. OSHA also requires that hepatitis B vaccines be available to all healthcare workers. OSHA develops and enforces standards of workplace safety and health. Workers may file a complaint with OSHA if the workplace is out of compliance.

15. B: If the phlebotomist is asked to transport a nonblood specimen, such as a urine sample, to the laboratory for testing, the phlebotomist should verify that the specimen is labeled correctly. The label should be on the container and not the lid (which must be removed for testing) and should contain the same type of identifying information as on the blood sample containers. Additionally, the type and source of the sample should be identified on the label because different types of samples may have similar appearances.

16. D: Collection timing is most critical for monitoring therapeutic drugs with short half-lives, such as the aminoglycosides. Timing is less critical for testing for levels of drugs with longer half-lives such as phenobarbital or digoxin, and even less so for ethanol, or blood alcohol, testing.

17. D: If a patient's test request requires a chemistry panel, a CBC, a PT, and blood typing, the order in which the specimens should be drawn is:

1. PT (light blue stopper)
2. Chemistry panel (red or gold stopper)
3. Blood typing (pink stopper)
4. CBC (lavender/purple stopper)

18. D: If protocol for blood C&S requires skin antisepsis with alcohol (70% isopropyl) followed by tincture of iodine (2%), but the patient is allergic to iodine, an acceptable alternate procedure is to wash the skin with soap and water, allow to dry, then cleanse twice with alcohol, allowing the skin to air dry after each cleansing. Skin asepsis is especially important with C&S because of the risk that skin bacteria will contaminate the specimen.

19. B: The parent of a minor has the legal right to receive information about the child's tests, so providing this information should not result in a lawsuit. However, doing a fingerstick on a 6-month-old infant increases the risk of injury to the bone, and only heelsticks should be done on children younger than 1 year. Misidentifying a patient could result in a lawsuit if harm comes to the patient as a result. Lowering a bed rail and leaving it down increases the risk of patient fall and injury.

20. D: The government agency responsible for regulations governing the use of gloves when carrying out a venipuncture is OSHA. These regulations are part of OSHA's Bloodborne Pathogen standards; the current version is part of the Needlestick Safety and Prevention Act (2000). This act was enacted to reduce the risk of needlestick injuries and blood contamination by healthcare workers and has promoted the use of safer medical devices and work practices. States may have their own OSHA-approved programs but must meet the minimum standards developed by OSHA.

21. B: Reflux of an additive is when the additive enters the needle and can therefore contaminate any tubes filled afterward. This may cause adverse effects if it occurs during venipuncture, especially if the additive is an anticoagulant such as EDTA, so the best method of preventing reflux is to place the arm in a downward position with the collection tube below the venipuncture site so that gravity prevents reflux. Care should also be taken to prevent back and forth movement of the tube during filling, as this mixes the specimen with the anticoagulant.

22. A: Bloodstained gauze should be disposed of in a biohazard waste container, not in a sharps container. All used needles and lancets should be placed in the sharps container. Any sharp should also be placed in the sharps container if the package is opened, even if the sharp is unused, because the purpose of the sharps container is to prevent both transmission of disease and trauma. Sharps containers are often red in color.

23. C: Rickets usually occurs in children and is marked by abnormal or "soft" bones. It is caused by a lack of vitamin D in the diet. Arthritis is an inflammatory condition of the joints, osteochondritis is an inflammation of the bone and cartilage, and osteomyelitis is inflammation of the bone or bone marrow caused by bacterial infection.

24. A: Steps that can help prevent the development of a hematoma include:

- Maintaining the position of the needle throughout the specimen collection
- Removing the tourniquet before removing the needle
- Removing the tube from the holder before removing the needle
- Examining the puncture site to ensure it is properly sealed prior to applying a bandage

142

If bruising, swelling, or other signs of a hematoma are evident during collection, the needle must be removed immediately and pressure must be applied to the site.

25. B: Asking a nurse (or anyone) to temporarily store a forensic specimen may violate the chain of custody. The phlebotomist obtaining the specimen should verify identification of the patient and clearly label the specimen, sign the chain of custody form, and place the specimen into a special transfer bag that is sealed, dated, and signed by the phlebotomist to ensure that the specimen has not been tampered with in any way.

26. D: A corrosive chemical is a health hazard as opposed to a physical hazard because contact with the chemical may result in health impairment, such as loss of tissue. Other health hazards include substances that are carcinogens (cancer-causing), irritants (e.g., eye or skin irritation), teratogens (birth defects), sensitizers (which cause an allergic response), and toxins (which can cause severe illness or death). Hazardous materials may be ingested orally, inhaled in fumes or aerosolized substances, or absorbed through the skin, eyes, or mucous membranes.

27. B: The percentage of total blood volume that can be collected from pediatric or critically ill patients is 1–5% within a 24-hour period, up to a total of 10% over an 8-week period. Therefore, it is important to estimate the patient's total blood volume and to monitor the volume of blood withdrawn in order to prevent iatrogenic anemia and/or hypovolemia. In some cases, it may be advisable to obtain capillary blood for tests to decrease the volume of blood needed, especially for young children.

28. C: If petechiae are noted on the patient's skin distal to the tourniquet, this suggests that the patient may have a coagulation defect, such as thrombocytopenia, and may have excessive bleeding after venipuncture. Other causes of petechiae can include medications (e.g., aspirin, anticoagulants) and some types of infectious/inflammatory disorders. Petechiae are nonraised lesions that are small (<3 mm) in diameter.

29. B: Hepatitis C virus (HCV) infection may occur through exposure to blood and serum and is primarily transmitted through sexual contact and needle sharing. However, it is rarely found in urine or semen and is not associated with phlebotomy procedures.

30. B: During venipuncture, if the needle appears to be in the vein but no blood is flowing and a slight vibration or quiver of the needle is noted, the most appropriate initial response is to remove the vacuum tube, pull back slightly on the needle, and reinsert the vacuum tube. If this is not successful, the venipuncture should be discontinued and another site attempted. The lack of blood flow and vibration or quiver suggest that the needle is in a valve and the valve is attempting to open and close.

31. A: If a venipuncture must be done at a specific time but the phlebotomist mistakenly collects the specimen 30 minutes late, the phlebotomist should report the late collection immediately because, depending on the type of test, the late collection may alter the results. If the situation is immediately brought to the attention of the laboratory supervisor, the specimen may be salvaged. It is unethical to fail to report an error or to hope that no one finds out.

32. A: The blood specimen for cold agglutinins must be maintained at body temperature through warming. Another test that requires the specimens to be warmed is cryoglobulin. Usually, the specimen is collected into tubes that are pre-warmed and then placed within 1 minute into a temperature-controlled environment, such as an insulated container with a water bath. The temperature should be maintained at 37 °C (98.6 °F) until the specimen is processed. Laboratory guidelines should always be consulted to ensure proper transport of specimens.

33. D: If the phlebotomist notes that a previous venipuncture site is tender and erythematous with a red streak extending 4 inches above the site, the likely cause is phlebitis, which is inflammation of the superficial veins, usually in the arms if associated with IVs or venipuncture. Phlebitis, which is associated with erythema, swelling, hardening of the vein, and tenderness, is usually not infective and often resolves with application of heat. However, if infection or deep vein thrombosis occurs, the symptoms spread, the patient is likely to run a fever, and pain may increase markedly.

34. A: The purpose of a Vein Entry Indicator Device (VEID) is to indicate when a needle penetrates a vein in order to increase the success rate for venipuncture, especially in individuals with small, fragile veins, those with excessive blood loss, and those with hard-to-locate veins. The needle is attached to a pressure-sensing device that notes the change in pressure when the needle penetrates a vein and emits a beep within a tenth of a second.

35. A: Serum that appears milky likely indicates lipemia, which is an increase in lipids (fats) from ingestion of foods high in fat, such as bacon, or from some intravenous feeding solutions. Lipemia may be evident for up to 12 hours after ingestion of a fatty food, so patients are asked to fast for 12 hours before tests on lipids, such as triglycerides, are performed. Additionally, lipemic serum may interfere with some chemistry tests.

36. B: In double-pointed needles, the rubber sheath that covers the shorter needle is intended to prevent leakage of blood when evacuated collection tubes are changed for multiple collections or when the final evacuated collection tube is removed. The sheath is retracted when a tube is pushed onto the needle to collect a sample and then covers the needle again as the tube is removed. This transfer needle is covered by a protective tube holder, which must be left in place for disposal.

37. D: Alcohol-based antisepsis is more commonly used than povidone-iodine–based antisepsis because povidone-iodine is more likely to cause an allergic response; many people are allergic to iodine. In most cases, the antiseptic of choice is 70% isopropyl alcohol in individually wrapped containers. Povidone-iodine has long been used for preparing sites for blood cultures and blood gases because it provides strong antisepsis, but its use is becoming less common. Other antiseptics include benzalkonium chloride, chlorhexidine gluconate, and hydrogen peroxide.

38. C: The collection tube cap color for specimens for PT (prothrombin time), aPTT (activated partial thromboplastin time), and TT (thrombin time) is light blue. All three tests must be done on plasma, and in all cases the collection tube must be filled to the correct volume. These three tests are often done together as screening for coagulation disorders. Normal values (which may vary slightly from one laboratory to another) are:

- PT: 10–13 seconds
- aPTT: 25–39 seconds
- TT: <20 seconds (usually 15–19)

39. A: The primary purpose of therapeutic drug monitoring (TDM) is to identify optimal dosing by monitoring blood levels of the drug at different time periods. Testing is often done when the medication peaks (highest blood level), which is usually 1–2 hours after oral medication, 1 hour after IM medication, or 30 minutes after IV medication. Testing is also done at the trough (lowest) level, which is usually about 15 minutes prior to the next scheduled dose.

40. B: If a patient is very thin and has prominent veins that require a low needle angle for venipuncture, the best choice is probably a winged ("butterfly") infusion set with a syringe because the syringe is not attached to the needle, so it does not get in the way. This allows for a very low angle for venipuncture as the needle can be held almost parallel to the skin. Most venipunctures are done at about a 30-degree angle, but each patient must be evaluated individually.

41. C: Venipuncture of the basilic vein, which runs along the ulnar side of the forearm, poses the greatest risk of accidental puncture of an artery because the vein lies in close proximity to the brachial artery. The median cubital vein is relatively large and less likely to roll than some other veins, so it is usually the first choice for venipuncture, followed by the cephalic vein, which lies on the radial side of the arm. The metacarpal veins are often easily visible, but should usually be avoided in older adults because they have little supporting subcutaneous tissue.

42. B: A patient lying on their stomach is in the prone position. A patient lying on their back, face up, is in the supine position. A patient standing erect with arms at their sides and palms facing forward is considered to be in the anatomic position. Reclined position is also referred to as semi-Fowler's position, with the head of the bed at approximately 30 to 45 degrees.

43. C: After a needle and tube holder are used to collect a blood specimen, the tube holder should be disposed of as one unit with the needle in the sharps container. Removing the tube holder is prohibited by OSHA because doing so increases the risk of needlestick injuries. Additionally, the tube holder may be contaminated with small particles of blood and cannot be reused or resterilized, so must be disposed of after use.

44. C: When asked to collect blood from a peripheral vascular access device, the phlebotomist should recognize that this procedure can only be performed if the phlebotomist has completed the required training, per facility protocol. The phlebotomist may often be asked to assist in the process of blood collection from a vascular access device by passing the appropriate tubes and advising about the volume of specimens needed and the order of draw. The filled collection tubes are usually transported to the lab by the phlebotomist.0

45. C: When loading a centrifuge that holds multiple tubes, if only one tube needs to be centrifuged, the phlebotomist should place the tube and a tube filled with the same volume of water across from it in the centrifuge. The centrifuge must be balanced. The tubes are filled with an equal volume and placed opposite each other to prevent vibration that may result in tubes being broken and samples aerosolized. If vibration occurs after the centrifuge is turned on, this often indicates an unbalanced load and requires that the centrifuge be immediately turned off.

46. B: If blood cannot be obtained from either arm, the phlebotomist must obtain a physician's order before using a foot or ankle for drawing blood,. Because circulation in the lower extremities is often impaired, using foot or ankle veins for blood specimens increases the risk of tissue necrosis, blood clots, and infection. If venipuncture in the foot or ankle is necessary, the phlebotomist should use a 22- or 23-gauge needle and a syringe rather than an evacuated collection tube to avoid causing the veins to collapse.

47. A: Normal blood glucose levels for a healthy adult should be in the range of 65–110 mg/dL.

48. C: When carrying out point-of-care (POC) testing for PT/INR with an analyzer such as the CoaguCheck XS Plus, a capillary blood drop should generally be applied to the test strip or other collection device within 15 seconds. A capillary tube may be used to collect the drop of blood and apply it to the test strip. The drop should be transferred by holding it near the test strip or collection device while avoiding touching or wiping the blood onto the strip or device.

49. B: Blood pressure cuffs require intermediate to low level disinfection, usually through wiping with a liquid disinfectant. While disinfection should destroy most (but not all) bacteria, viruses, and fungi, it does not destroy bacterial spores. Surgical instruments require sterilization, which destroys all microorganisms as well as bacterial spores. Cleaning, on the other hand, is all that is generally needed for windows and furniture in a waiting area where people who are clothed have sat.

50. D: The Occupational Safety and Health Administration (OSHA) requires that a high-efficiency particulate air (HEPA) respirator be used to protect healthcare workers caring for acid-fast-bacilli (AFB) patients, such as those with infectious tuberculosis. A HEPA respirator is not required for enteric or contact isolation patients or caring for burn patients.

51. D: When using an evacuated tube system for venipuncture, the phlebotomist must rely on sensing a decrease in resistance to determine if the needle is correctly positioned in the vein. There is no flash of blood with an evacuated tube system, only with a needle and syringe. If the phlebotomist notes that the needle is vibrating, this is an indication that the needle is in a valve and needs to be repositioned. No blood will flow into the holder until the vacuum tube is inserted.

52. B: OSHA requires that employers provide healthcare workers with the appropriate PPE (personal protective equipment) at no cost so that they can perform their job functions safely without risk of infection or injury. PPE may vary according to the job description and situation, but available PPE should include gloves, masks, face shields, shoe coverings, hair coverings, protective gowns, and N-95 respirators. Additional PPE is required for those caring for Ebola patients.

53. D: If a laboratory detects a suspected outbreak of an infectious disease, such as *E. coli* infections, the laboratory should report this to their local or state health department. The health department will investigate and then report their findings to the Centers for Disease Control and Prevention (CDC) through the National Outbreak Reporting System (NORS). The CDC may take action depending on the information reported through NORS and their own investigations. The CDC maintains the Global Health Center, the goal of which is to protect the health and safety of Americans by tracking disease outbreaks and ensuring efforts to reduce disease incidence worldwide. The CDC monitors outbreaks throughout the world, takes measures to prevent spread, and provides technical assistance to public health organizations worldwide, often in conjunction with the World Health Organization.

54. B: Before a blood specimen is collected from a newborn for routine screening for inborn errors of metabolism (IEM), the infant should have nursed or been bottle-fed for at least 24 hours (48 is optimal) because many IEMs are related to problems with protein metabolism; therefore, the child needs to ingest protein in order for the test results to be accurate. Because some mothers and infants are discharged within 24 hours and the tests may not be completely accurate, all mothers should be advised of the importance of a repeat screening after discharge.

55. D: The primary use of non-additive evacuated plastic collection tubes is for discard tubes when a few milliliters of blood must be discarded prior to collection of the sample. If, for example, a winged infusion set ("butterfly") is used to draw a blood sample, which is to be collected in a light-blue–capped (citrate) evacuated tube, a discard tube must be used first to ensure that all dead space in the needle and tubing is filled with blood before the sample is collected to make sure the ratio of blood to additive is correct.

56. A: Cotton balls should not be used to apply alcohol to the skin because small particles of cotton lint may adhere to the skin and be injected during venipuncture. Alcohol pads and/or povidone-iodine wipes should be used for skin antisepsis. Other equipment needed for routine venipuncture includes evacuated collection tubes, a tourniquet, lint-free gauze, tape or stretch nonadhesive bandages, gloves, and syringes.

57. B: If blood must be drawn from an arm with an IV in place, the phlebotomist should ask the nurse to turn off the IV and then wait at least 2 minutes before attempting venipuncture to decrease the dilution of the blood. The phlebotomist is not allowed to adjust or stop the flow of an IV. A tourniquet must be applied distal to the IV, and the venipuncture is carried out distal to the tourniquet. The phlebotomist should record the type of fluid and medication (if applicable) in the IV. The phlebotomist must notify the nurse that the venipuncture is complete and the IV needs to be restarted.

58. C: The evacuated collection tube that cannot be used to collect a specimen for a BMP is the lavender-capped collection tube, which contains an anticoagulant (EDTA) and is used to collect a whole blood sample for the CBC or its components. Red-capped collection tubes with a clot activator, red/black SST, and green-capped tubes can all be used. The BMP includes the tests on the electrolyte panel as well as the BUN, Ca (calcium), creatinine, and glucose.

59. A: An electrolyte panel includes HCO_3 (bicarbonate), Cl (chloride), K (potassium), and Na (sodium), amongst others. Tests can be done using either plasma or serum. Evacuated collection tubes that can be used for the electrolyte panel include red top, red/black-top SST (serum separator tube), and green top. If the collection tube contains a clot activator, it should be inverted a minimum of 5 times. If the collection tube contains lithium heparin, an anticoagulant, it should be inverted at least 8 times.

60. B: Physician office laboratories are most often accredited by COLA (Commission on Laboratory Accreditation), which was founded in 1988 with the original intent of inspecting and accrediting physician office laboratories to ensure that they are in compliance with CLIA (Clinical Laboratory Improvement Amendments). COLA has since expanded its mission and now also accredits hospital laboratories and independent laboratories. CMS (Centers for Medicare and Medicaid Services) and The Joint Commission have granted deeming authority to COLA.

61. D: For venipuncture, the vein should be anchored distal to the puncture site, safely out of reach of the tip of the needle by 1–2 inches. The thumb of the free hand is used to anchor the vein with a downward pull so that the skin is taut. The vein should not be anchored on either side or proximal to the puncture site because this increases the risk of accidental needlestick injury and may impede acquisition of the blood sample.

62. A: The tests that are typically available on a point-of-care (POC) arterial blood gas (ABG) analyzer include the following:

- pH: acidity/alkalinity
- TCO_2: total carbon dioxide, including intermediate forms
- PO_2: partial pressure of dissolved oxygen in the blood
- PCO_2: partial pressure of dissolved carbon dioxide in the blood
- SO_2: percentage of hemoglobin-binding sites in the blood occupied by oxygen
- HCO_3: concentration of hydrogen carbonate (a by-product of metabolism) in the blood
- Base excess/deficit: excess with metabolic alkalosis and deficit with metabolic acidosis

63. C: When carrying out a heelstick blood collection on a newborn, the depth of the puncture should be equal to or less than 2 mm. In a newborn, the blood supply is typically located 0.35–1.6 mm below the skin. Thus, a 2 mm depth provides an adequate flow of blood but is generally too shallow to cause injury to the calcaneus. The heelstick should be done on the lateral aspects of the heel rather than the middle or posterior aspects to ensure that the calcaneus is avoided.

64. A: The stopper color that indicates the correct tube for a complete blood count (CBC) is lavender/purple (EDTA). This tube is used for CBC, differential, reticulocyte count, sedimentation (sed) rate, platelet count, Coombs test, cyclosporine test, and flow cytometry. The light-blue-top tube (3.2% sodium citrate) is used for coagulation tests such as PT, PTT, and thrombin clotting time. The pink-top tube (K_2EDTA) is used for blood typing and screening, direct Coombs, and HIV viral load. The green-top tube (sodium heparin) is used for ammonia, lactate, and human leukocyte antigen typing.

65. C: For venipuncture, the vein that should always be selected as the last option is the basilic vein because it lies near the brachial artery, so accidental arterial puncture may occur. Additionally, nerves run parallel to the basilic vein, increasing the risk of injury to the nerve. The order in which the veins should be inspected is: median cubital, cephalic, basilic, dorsal metacarpal, and wrist. For venipuncture, the basilic vein goes to the end of the list.

66. B: The order in which pediatric micro-collection containers differs from the standard order of draw used with evacuated tubes. For micro-collection containers, the correct order is lavender (which contains EDTA anticoagulant), green (which contains sodium or lithium heparin), and finally red (which does not contain additives). The lavender tube is used for standard hematology tests (such as RBC and WBC counts), which are often most important, so it should be collected first to ensure that the volume collected is adequate, since obtaining adequate amounts of blood from pediatric patients can be difficult.

67. B: In administering a tuberculosis (TB) skin test, the antigen should be injected just below the skin, not into a vein. Presence of a bleb, or wheal, indicates that the antigen was injected properly. A TB reaction is measured according to the degree of induration (hardness), not erythema (redness).

68. D: If a gray-capped collection tube, which is used for glucose testing, is overfilled, the result may be clotting of the specimen because overfilling results in an inadequate amount of additive needed to inactivate clotting. Therefore, the specimen must be discarded. Underfilling a gray-capped collection tube, on the other hand, causes a dilution effect, and the excess additive may result in low test results. The minimum draw volume is 50% of capacity.

69. A: The Clinical and Laboratory Standards Institute (CLSI) provides standards for a wide range of performance and testing and covers all types of laboratory functions, including microbiology. The institute comprises representatives from the healthcare professions, industry, and government. These standards are used as a basis for quality control procedures. Standards include labeling, security/information technology, toxicology/drug testing, statistical quality control, and performance standards for various types of antimicrobial susceptibility testing.

70. B: If venipuncture is required for an elderly patient with obvious tremors of the upper extremities, the best solution is to ask a nurse to assist in stabilizing the arm. Equipment should be chosen carefully to avoid unnecessary trauma and prolonged venipuncture. Older adults, especially those with small, friable veins, may bruise easily. Nonadhesive elastic bandaging may be more appropriate than adhesive bandages because of the thinness of skin in older adults.

71. B: The vein-finder device that projects a pattern map of the veins on the skin is the near-infrared light device. The device is held above the skin, and the veins are outlined on the skin surface as the veins absorb the infrared light and the infrared light is reflected off of the other tissue. Infrared vein finders are available in mounted (for hands-free use) or handheld versions. The devices are especially useful with patients who have poorly visible veins and/or dark skin.

72. B: Sputum specimens should ideally be obtained first thing in the morning upon arising because patients tend to cough up secretions that have pooled during the night, so it is easier to get a large volume of sputum. Sputum should be obtained at least 1 hour after eating so it is not contaminated with food particles or vomitus. Before obtaining the specimen, the patient should be asked to remove dentures and to thoroughly rinse the mouth with water and gargle to reduce contaminants.

73. D: If a very small hematoma is evident during venipuncture, the best initial response is to observe the site and complete the venipuncture. If, however, the hematoma is large or expanding, then the phlebotomist should remove the needle, elevate the arm above the level of the heart, and apply pressure until the bleeding stops. Small hematomas are fairly common, especially in patients taking anticoagulants and certain other drugs, as well as older adults, whose veins may be friable.

74. A: The greatest risk when a tube breaks during centrifugation is aerosolization of the specimen because the spinning specimen breaks down into droplets, which can be easily inhaled or can land on exposed skin, increasing risk of infection. Aerosolization can also occur if collection tubes are overfilled or if the caps come off during processing. Additionally, care must be used if removing a cap after centrifugation. Buckets, tubes, and rotors should be carefully spaced and balanced before centrifugation.

75. A: For forensic collection of a blood sample, the specimen container must be placed and sealed inside a transfer bag. Careful documentation regarding patient identification and date and time of venipuncture is critical to establish the chain of custody. The phlebotomist signs the transfer form and the transfer bag (if a signature is required) to indicate that the chain of custody has not been breached. The bag must remain sealed until it is processed by the appropriate laboratory.

76. B: According to the Americans with Disabilities Act (ADA), to ensure accessibility to patients on crutches or in wheelchairs, at least one space next to the phlebotomy chair must have a minimum area of 30 × 48 inches. Space should be available for a wheelchair to turn 180°. There must be adequate space on either side of the phlebotomy chair for transfers to and from gurneys, wheelchairs, or stretchers, and both sides must allow access to the patient. A bariatric phlebotomy chair should be available for large patients.

77. B: When the phlebotomist is using microcollection tubes for a fingerstick, the collection tube that should usually be filled first is the lavender-capped tube (this different from the order used with venipuncture) to ensure that the volume collected is sufficient for hematology tests. This is followed by other collection tubes that contain additives, and the plain tubes utilized for serum collection are filled last. In most cases, the first drop of blood is wiped away and the second drop of blood is collected.

78. C: When collecting a capillary blood specimen for bilirubin from a newborn receiving phototherapy for jaundice, it is especially important to turn off the phototherapy light during collection because exposure of the blood sample to the light may break down the bilirubin. The specimen must be obtained carefully to prevent hemolysis and placed in an amber microcollection container, or the container should be covered with aluminum foil to protect the contents from light. The blood specimen should be collected as soon after the request as possible because accurate timing can help to determine the rate of bilirubin increase.

79. B: The correct method of removing a stopper from a specimen tube is to pull it straight up and away from the tube. If possible, a removal device or robotics should be used to minimize human contact. Any fluid in contact with the stopper may become aerosolized when the stopper is removed; therefore, if a tube does not have a built-in safety feature to prevent aerosolization, the stopper should be grasped with a gauze pad or a tissue.

80. B: The billing code system that is used for laboratory testing for inpatients is ICD-10-PCS (International Classification of Diseases, 10th Revision, Procedure Coding System). It is used to report and bill procedures while patients are hospitalized. Outpatient procedures, on the other hand, are billed using CPT (Current Procedural Terminology) codes. ICD-11 (International Classification of Diseases, 11th Revision) is the latest code system for diagnoses, but it has yet to be adopted in the US. The ICD-10-CM (International Classification of Diseases, 10th Revision, Clinical Modification) is still the coding system used in the US for documenting a diagnosis.

81. C: If the phlebotomist drops an unused glass collection tube, causing it to break and scatter pieces of glass, the phlebotomist should guard the area to prevent anyone from being injured and call housekeeping. The glass should be removed with a brush and dustpan. Any large pieces should be picked up with forceps or tongs and never picked up by hand because this can result in lacerations. Whenever possible, plastic containers and collection tubes should be used instead of glass to minimize risk from breakage.

82. D: Iodophors take 90–120 seconds to adequately disinfect the skin for blood cultures. The usual procedure is to cleanse the skin with a 30-second friction rub with 70% isopropyl alcohol, allow the alcohol to dry completely, then apply the main disinfectant and let it dry for the time recommended by the manufacturer. If the phlebotomist needs to palpate the vein after applying the disinfectant, sterile gloves must be worn.

83. D: Metal filings ("fleas") may be used with capillary blood gas collection tubes to mix blood with the anticoagulant in the tube. They are inserted into the tube and serve as stirrers. Capillary blood gas collection tubes are long and thin and commonly hold up to 100 µL of blood. A band around the tube identifies the additive; most commonly, this is a green band indicating the additive sodium heparin. A magnet may also be used to mix the specimen. The magnet fits over the tube and is slid up and down the length of the tube.

84. A: Blood gas values, such as partial pressure of carbon dioxide (pCO_2), are typically ordered STAT. Human chorionic gonadotropin (hCG) is a pregnancy test. The fasting blood sugar (FBS) test is a timed test for which patients must restrict dietary intake for 12 hours. The hemoglobin (Hgb) test is used to diagnose anemia.

85. D: The Joint Commission is primarily an accrediting organization for healthcare facilities and programs nationally and internationally. The Joint Commission accredits hospitals, critical access hospitals, ambulatory care centers, behavioral healthcare programs, home care services (which include hospices and pharmacies), laboratories (hospital-based and freestanding), and nursing care centers. The Joint Commission also offers a number of certificates (e.g., palliative care, disease-specific care, staffing, integrated care, and primary care medical home), which indicate that a program has met specific standards.

86. B: The phlebotomist should evaluate the risk of violence with all patients. While some patients may show outward signs of impending violence, such as by making threatening gestures or using abusive language, others (such as patients with dementia) may seem outwardly calm but react violently to venipuncture. If the phlebotomist fears violence, they should make sure that the exit is clear and that another staff person is in attendance to help if necessary. The phlebotomist should remain calm and speak in a soothing manner.

87. D: When opening and aliquoting a specimen, the required PPE includes gown, gloves, and face shield. Otherwise, the opening must occur behind a portable splash screen that is placed between the specimen and the person's body. The sample should be removed from the tube with a disposable pipette and placed into the aliquot tube. Pouring the specimen from the specimen tube into the aliquot tube must be avoided because this may result in aerosolization.

88. D: Blood draws for a GTT (glucose tolerance test) in pregnancy, which is done to screen for gestational diabetes, are usually done at 1 hour, 2 hours, and 3 hours after the test begins. Prior to beginning the timed portion of the test, a FBS (fasting blood sugar) is checked to ensure that the level is within a safe range. If so, the patient drinks the glucose solution within 5 minutes and the timed period of the test begins. The patient should be advised to eat no food and only drink water during the testing period. There are other variations of the GTT that require different testing intervals.

89. A: When using a pediatric vein transilluminator with an infant, the transilluminator should be placed in the palm of the child's hand. The light projects through the hand and helps the phlebotomist locate the veins in the hand. Adult transilluminators are held onto the skin and project light downward to help illuminate the veins. The adult device has a horseshoe shape, so it can illuminate the veins from three sides. Transilluminators require a second person to hold the device in place during the venipuncture.

90. D: Blood must be drawn from an artery for blood gases. Because arteries tend to be deeper, have thicker walls, and be in closer proximity to nerves, withdrawing blood from arteries is more difficult than from veins and must be done by someone trained to do the procedure, such as an RN, when it is within the person's scope of practice. Additionally, arterial blood draws, usually done in the wrist, are more painful than venous blood draws and may result in bleeding, hematoma, ecchymosis, and infection.

91. C: According to CLSI guidelines on the venous blood specimen collection process, the first step in carrying out a venipuncture is to identify the patient. Proper identification procedure requires the use of two identifiers. In a laboratory setting, this usually involves verifying the patient's name and birthdate by asking the patient for the information rather than providing the information and asking if it is correct. In an inpatient facility, the patient should always be asked to give his or her name and birthdate if the patient is cognizant, and the name band should be checked as well for the name and identification number. The patient is then provided information on the procedure (including the purpose) and consent is obtained. After the phlebotomist conducts appropriate hand hygiene, the patient is then assessed for possible complications and positioned in a reclining or seated position, the site for the venipuncture is identified, and the specimen is collected.

92. B: While *Mycobacterium tuberculosis* is highly infectious, better treatment and early diagnosis have markedly decreased incidence, so it is rarely a cause of nosocomial infections unless a patient has been misdiagnosed. Three common pathogenic agents associated with nosocomial (healthcare-associated) infections are *Klebsiella pneumoniae*; *Staphylococcus aureus*, particularly MRSA (methicillin-resistant *Staphylococcus aureus*); and *Clostridioides difficile*. *Klebsiella pneumoniae* can cause antibiotic-resistant infections. *Staphylococcus aureus* is often associated with wound and soft tissue infections. *Clostridioides difficile* results in infection of the GI system and severe diarrhea.

93. A: In the United States, all laboratory testing, except for research, is regulated by Centers for Medicare and Medicaid Services (CMS) through the Clinical Laboratory Improvement Amendments (CLIA). CLIA is implemented through the Division of Laboratory Services and serves approximately 244,000 laboratories. Laboratories receiving reimbursement from CMS must meet CLIA standards, which ensure that laboratory testing will be accurate and procedures followed properly. The CDC partners with CMS and the Food and Drug Administration (FDA) in supporting CLIA programs.

94. D: If the phlebotomist observes another worker placing needles and syringes into a personal bag before leaving work, the best response is to notify a supervisor as soon as possible, describing the observation in detail. Confronting another person who is doing an illegal or unethical act may precipitate a violent response. Most organizations have established protocols for dealing with theft, and the supervisor should determine whether the police should be called.

95. C: The urine culture and sensitivity (C&S) test is used to identify the bacteria or fungus that caused a urinary tract infection (UTI) and the medications that can successfully treat the UTI. An ACTH test is used to assess adrenocorticotropic hormone. A TSH test is used to assess thyroid-stimulating hormone levels. FBS is the fasting blood sugar test.

96. C: Body position, environmental conditions such as temperature and humidity, and stress can affect blood specimen composition. Fasting is useful in eliminating dietary influences on blood testing.

97. A: Separated serum or plasma specimens should be maintained at room temperature for no more than 2 hours. This maximum time limit is used because it complies with the requirements for numerous tests, including glucose, lactate dehydrogenase, catecholamines, lactic acid, and potassium. Processing a specimen within this time frame prevents further metabolic changes, such as glycolysis, that may affect the test results.

98. D: If an indwelling line, such as a central venous catheter, is used to obtain a blood sample, 5 mL of blood should be discarded before the sample of blood is collected in order to clear the sample of any intravenous fluids or medications that were administered through the central venous line. In some cases, the initial blood withdrawn is readministered to the patient after the specimen is obtained in order to prevent iatrogenic anemia.

99. B: Bilirubin is normally present in blood, but not in urine; the presence of bilirubin in urine is indicative of liver or gallbladder disease or cancer. Albumin is the primary protein found in urine. Ketones are end products of fat metabolism and normally present in urine. Bacteria may be present in urine in small amounts; only large quantities of bacteria are indicative of pathology.

100. A: If the phlebotomist is asked to draw blood from a hospitalized patient who has lost her armband, the phlebotomist's first action should be to ask staff to replace the armband. The phlebotomist should not draw blood on any hospitalized patient unless an armband is present. Patients in the emergency department should be assigned a temporary unique identifier (such as a patient number). Outpatients do not require armbands but the phlebotomist should verify that the patient's name and birthdate or other identifying information matches that on the laboratory request forms.

101. A: A test request should include the following specific information about the patient:

- Name: first, middle, last
- Identification (ID)/Record number
- Gender: male or female (typically the gender assigned at birth, but this may vary if the patient is nonbinary or transgender)
- Date of birth

In addition to information about the patient, the test request should include the name of the ordering healthcare provider, the tests to be performed, the collection site (if appropriate), the date the collection is to be made, and any additional instructions that are necessary.

102. A: If a patient is very angry and yells that the lab tests are a "waste of time," the best initial response is to stay calm and listen, allowing the patient to vent. Patients are often frustrated, frightened, and in pain, and these factors may cause patients to lash out at those caring for them. Once the patient has expressed his or her feelings and calmed somewhat, the phlebotomist should speak calmly, expressing empathy and using the patient's name to personalize the exchange.

103. D: If a patient has paralysis and lack of sensation in the right arm and hand, the best choice for venipuncture is any appropriate site on the left arm. With paralysis, muscle tone is lost, and this may cause some pooling of blood, increasing the risk of thromboses. Additionally, the lack of sensation means that if a nerve is inadvertently injured, the patient will be unaware. If venipuncture from a paralyzed limb cannot be avoided, then the phlebotomist should follow procedures carefully and avoid any lateral probing and ensure that pressure is held on the puncture site until any bleeding has stopped.

104. C: When transporting a specimen at room temperature, an appropriate temperature is 22° C (71.6 °F). Specimens that are transported or handled at room temperature should be maintained in an environment around 20–30 °C (68–86 °F), although some measurands may begin to deteriorate with extended temperatures greater than 22 °C (71.6 °F). Specimens that must be maintained at body temperature should be kept at 36.4–37.6 °C (96.8–99.7 °F). Specimens transported and handled in the wrong temperature range may be altered.

105. B: If a patient is chewing gum when the phlebotomist arrives to collect a blood specimen, the phlebotomist should ask the patient to remove the gum before proceeding. The patient should not be eating or drinking anything or have anything in the mouth, except for what is needed for medical treatment. Because patients sometimes jerk or even faint during venipuncture, they may choke on the gum or other substance or swallow it inadvertently.

106. A: When using an evacuated tube system for venipuncture, the phlebotomist can determine that a tube is properly filled when the vacuum is exhausted. Each type of tube has a vacuum that will provide the volume necessary for getting the correct ratio of blood to the tube additive (if any) and the tests that may be run on the sample. Typical volumes are 2.0–8.5 mL. The tube should also be examined after filling to ensure that it appears to contain the correct volume.

107. C: If a phlebotomist sustains a needlestick injury, the first step is to immediately wash the puncture site with soap and water. As soon as possible, the supervisor should be notified and the injury reported according to protocol. The patient source should be identified so that they can be tested for HIV, HBV, and HCV with consent. The phlebotomist should report to the designated health service so that testing procedures can be outlined and PEP (post-exposure prophylaxis) started if necessary.

108. C: Using a foot vein for a blood draw increases risk of blood clots because circulation is often impaired in the legs and feet, especially in older and/or diabetic patients. Patients are also at increased risk of ulceration of the site. Drawing blood from the foot or ankle should be avoided, but if neither arm can be used, blood may be drawn from the foot or ankle with a physician's order.

109. A: When drawing a blood specimen from an adolescent, the phlebotomist should recognize that most adolescents are self-conscious and concerned about their bodies and appearance. They may become embarrassed easily, so it is important that their privacy be maintained. Some may be afraid to express their fears in an attempt to "act like an adult," while others may act belligerently to hide fears. The phlebotomist should explain the procedure completely and ask if the patient has questions.

110. B: The preferred capillary puncture site for adults and children older than 1 year of age is the distal segment of the nondominant third or fourth finger (palmar surface). The nondominant hand tends to be less calloused than the dominant hand. The tip of the finger should be avoided, and the puncture should be made perpendicular to whorls. Capillary blood should not be obtained on the same side as a prior mastectomy without written permission of the physician.

111. B: The chain of custody for a blood specimen, such as one for drug testing, begins with the initial contact with the patient when the venipuncture is carried out. A chain of custody form or other record should be filled out, and information is entered with each specimen transfer from the initial one until the final disposition. Each person involved must be identified and must sign or initialize the form/record, and each process carried out on the sample must be described. The sample must be stored in a secured and restricted storage site.

112. D: The non-profit organization CLSI (Clinical and Laboratory Standards Institute) determines the order of draw and publishes this information in the publication *Procedures for the Collection of Diagnostic Blood Specimens*, which is updated periodically to reflect changes in the healthcare industry and findings related to research. Hospitals and other healthcare organizations should use the current order of draw unless they have evidence-based research that supports altering this order. Some newer tubes are not listed in the order of draw, so the manufacturer's directions regarding order should be followed.

113. A: The abbreviation for the thyroid hormone triiodothyronine is T_3. It is the active form of thyroxine. The T_3 level increases with hyperthyroidism and decreases with hypothyroidism. T_4 is the abbreviation for thyroxine; TSH is thyroid stimulating hormone; and TBG is thyroxine-binding globulin. Orders for tests with similar abbreviations should always be double-checked to ensure that the correct blood sample is obtained and the correct test is conducted.

114. A: Removing the stoppers from blood specimen tubes during the precentrifugation period can result in an increase—not a decrease—of pH because of a loss of carbon dioxide (CO_2). Other problems that may occur if a stopper is removed are due to evaporation of the specimen, which can result in concentration and possibly alter the test results. An opened specimen container also always runs the risk of contamination. Containers should be maintained in an upright position with the stoppers in place.

115. A: Because outpatient specimens are not obtained during the basal state, normal values may differ slightly from those of inpatients. Hemoglobin (Hgb), hematocrit (Hct), and red blood cell (RBC) counts may have higher normal ranges at higher elevations. Caffeinated beverages may affect cortisol levels. Ingestion of lipids (fats) such as butter or cheese may increase blood lipid content, giving blood specimens a cloudy or milky appearance.

116. C: A blood sample in a gray-capped evacuated collection tube should be inverted a minimum of 8 times to ensure that the additive mixes adequately with the blood specimen. The gray-capped collection tube is used for glucose testing. Additives can include potassium oxalate/sodium fluoride, sodium fluoride only, or sodium fluoride/Na_2EDTA. Because glucose levels vary with food intake, patients usually fast for 8 hours prior to testing unless the order specifically indicates times, such as after meals.

117. D: The closure cap of the collection tube that contains sodium citrate is light blue. Sodium citrate is an anticoagulant, and the cap is color-coded so the phlebotomist can easily identify the correct tube. The light-blue–capped tube is utilized when conducting anticoagulant tests (PT, PTT, TT, and coagulation factors) on plasma because the anticoagulant prevents coagulation from occurring before the specimen is processed. It is important to fill the light-blue–capped evacuated tubes to capacity because the results may be inaccurate if they are not filled completely.

118. A: If a coagulation test requires platelet-poor plasma, it is necessary to centrifuge the specimen, use a pipette to carefully remove three-quarters of the plasma at the surface (avoid pouring), place it into an aliquot tube, and then centrifuge the aliquot tube to separate any remaining cells. Then, the plasma from the second centrifugation is transferred via a new pipette into another new tube for testing. Because platelets contain clotting factors, it is essential to remove platelets before carrying out the tests. Platelet-poor plasma should have fewer than 10,000 platelets/μL.

119. D: Blood cultures cannot be carried out on a specimen obtained through heelstick or other capillary samples because there is a potential for contamination and because blood cultures require large volumes of blood. Coagulation studies also cannot be carried out with a capillary sample. Capillary samples can only be used if a small quantity of blood is necessary. Tests that can be carried out using capillary samples include most chemistries, CBC, blood gas analysis, toxicology tests, liver function tests, and newborn screening. Capillary collection may be used for infants as well as adults.

120. C: For the C-urea breath test, used to detect *Helicobacter pylori* infection (a common cause of stomach and duodenal ulcers), the patient exhales into a Mylar balloon for a baseline breath sample and then drinks a solution containing synthetic urea, which contains carbon-13. A second exhalation sample is then obtained 15 minutes after the patient ingests the solution. If *H. pylori* is present, it will metabolize the synthetic urea and release CO_2 containing the carbon-13, which can be detected in the breath sample.

Practice Test #3

1. Which of the following governmental agencies or policies governs the accommodations that must be made in the laboratory for patients and workers who use wheelchairs?

    a. FDA
    b. ADHQ
    c. ADA
    d. EMTALA

2. Which type of fire extinguisher can be used to put out an electrical fire?

    a. Type A (water)
    b. Type AB (foam)
    c. Type D (dry metal power)
    d. Type ABC (ammonium phosphate)

3. Which of the following conditions can be caused by dysfunction of the pituitary gland?

    a. Cushing syndrome
    b. Dwarfism
    c. Diabetes
    d. Parkinson's disease

4. A specimen for a bilirubin test should be:

    a. Processed within 15 minutes
    b. Maintained at body temperature
    c. Protected from light
    d. Chilled immediately

5. If a patient continuously rubs her hands together and licks her lips when the phlebotomist is explaining a procedure, the phlebotomist should consider that the patient is likely:

    a. Dehydrated
    b. Nervous
    c. Angry
    d. In pain

6. he maximum size of syringe that should be used for blood collection is:

    a. 5 mL
    b. 10 mL
    c. 20 mL
    d. 50 mL

7. If a specimen must be refrigerated, the temperature should range from:

    a. 0–1 °C (32–33.8 °F)
    b. 2–10 °C (35.6–50 °F)
    c. 4–12 °C (39.2–53.6 °F)
    d. 2–15 °C (41–59 °F)

8. According to CLSI standards, the phlebotomist should wear _____ while inside the laboratory.

  a. a long-sleeved laboratory coat/gown
  b. a clean uniform
  c. isolation gear
  d. gloves and a mask

9. In performing the Allen test:

  a. The patient should hyperextend the fingers.
  b. Blanching of the hand indicates a positive result.
  c. Both the radial and ulnar arteries should be compressed at the same time.
  d. Only the radial artery should be compressed.

10. According to the order of the draw for venous blood, which of the following tubes is always drawn first?

  a. Light blue (3.2% sodium citrate)
  b. Blood cultures
  c. Green (sodium heparin)
  d. Pink (K_2EDTA)

11. With outpatients, urine specimens should be collected prior to venipuncture because:

  a. Patients may feel lightheaded and faint after venipuncture.
  b. Patients may forget about the urine specimen and leave.
  c. Blood in the urine may indicate the risk of excess bleeding.
  d. Patients may have more difficulty urinating after venipuncture.

12. The HIV test is an example of which type of laboratory test?

  a. Immunologic
  b. Chemical
  c. Microbiologic
  d. Coagulation

13. Phlebotomists are most likely to develop sensitivity to latex because of:

  a. Exposure to latex tourniquets
  b. Wearing latex gloves
  c. Cross-reactivity to food allergies
  d. Exposure to latex-capped collection tubes

14. Which of the following tests is included in a hepatic function panel?

  a. Albumin
  b. Creatine kinase
  c. ESR
  d. Cryoglobulin

15. When collecting blood specimens with collection tubes, the first three closure tops, according to the order of draw, (first to last) are:

    a. Yellow, light blue, and gold
    b. Yellow, light blue, and red
    c. Red, light blue, and yellow
    d. Gold, red, and green

16. According to the American Hospital Association's *The Patient Care Partnership*, patients do NOT have the right to expect:

    a. A clean, safe environment
    b. Privacy protection
    c. Cost-effective care
    d. Involvement in care

17. An individual with which type of blood can be a blood donor to individuals with any of the four blood types?

    a. Type A
    b. Type B
    c. Type AB
    d. Type O

18. The organization that develops and publishes the National Patient Safety Goals is:

    a. The Joint Commission
    b. COLA
    c. CAP
    d. CLIA

19. When performing venipuncture on a patient with small, fragile veins, the best solution is to use a:

    a. Winged infusion set with syringe
    b. Winged infusion set with evacuated tube
    c. Small-sized needle with evacuated tube
    d. Standard-sized needle with evacuated tube

20. When entering a room to draw blood from an individual on contact precautions, which PPE is generally required?

    a. Gloves only
    b. Gloves and gown
    c. Gloves, gown, and face shield
    d. Gloves, gown, face shield, and respirator

21. When collecting a sample of whole blood for testing using a lavender-capped microcollection tube, how many inversions are needed to mix the blood with the additive?

    a. 3–4
    b. 5–10
    c. 8–10
    d. 10–12

22. If a hospital laboratory is accredited by CAP, how frequently is the accreditation reviewed?

    a. Annually
    b. Every 2 years
    c. Every 3 years
    d. Every 4 years

23. The outermost layer of the skin is known as the:

    a. Dermis
    b. Epidermis
    c. Subcutaneous layer
    d. Hypodermal layer

24. A phlebotomist underfilled one collection tube (tube A) and overfilled another (tube B). If both tubes have the same additive, what is the best method to remedy the situation?

    a. Transfer some blood from tube B to tube A.
    b. Redraw blood for both tubes.
    c. Redraw for tube A.
    d. Redraw for tube B.

25. If the laboratory institutes policy and procedural changes, the phlebotomist should:

    a. Expect to be consulted.
    b. Expect to receive a salary increase.
    c. Expect to receive appropriate training.
    d. Expect to evaluate the procedures.

26. Postexposure vaccination is recommended for:

    a. Influenza B
    b. Measles
    c. HIV
    d. Pertussis

27. The C-hold (anchoring the vein with the index finger above the venipuncture site and the thumb below):

    a. Is used for rolling veins
    b. Increases risk of needlestick
    c. May collapse the vein
    d. Is an advanced technique

28. Which of the following is a form of arthritis?

    a. Bursitis
    b. Gout
    c. Rickets
    d. Slipped disc

29. The cap color for the collection tube used for tests of therapeutic drug levels is:
   a. Gold
   b. Green
   c. Light blue
   d. Gray

30. Which veins should NOT be used for venipuncture?
   a. Veins on the dorsal side of the hand
   b. Veins on the palmar side of the hand
   c. Veins on the dorsal side of the wrist
   d. Veins in the forearm

31. The proper use of a disinfectant is on:
   a. Skin
   b. Inanimate objects
   c. Mucous membranes
   d. Skin and inanimate objects

32. If a patient complains of feeling faint during collection of a blood specimen, the tourniquet and needle should be removed, pressure should be applied, and then the patient should be:
   a. Provided an ammonia inhalant
   b. Encouraged to take deep breaths
   c. Reclined, lain flat, or the head and arms lowered
   d. Provided with oxygen

33. After a blood specimen is collected in a tube that contains EDTA, the tube should be inverted:
   a. 3–4 times
   b. 5–10 times
   c. 8–10 times
   d. 10–12 times

34. A preservative used in the laboratory is categorized as which type of hazard?
   a. Biologic
   b. Chemical
   c. Physical
   d. Explosive

35. Which of the following statements regarding obtaining a blood specimen from a patient is FALSE?
   a. The phlebotomist should ask the patient's permission before collecting blood.
   b. The patient has the right to refuse the blood draw.
   c. The name of the ordering physician on the ID band should not differ from that on the requisition form.
   d. Patient identity should always be verified.

36. Which of the following is NOT a violation of general laboratory safety rules?

a. Wearing a laboratory coat when leaving the lab
b. Wearing nail polish
c. Wearing large earrings
d. Having shoulder-length hair

37. Evacuated collection tubes can be stored at:

a. Any temperature
b. 1–20 °C
c. 4–25 °C
d. 18–25 °C

38. The C-urea breath test is used to detect:

a. Lactose intolerance
b. *H. pylori* infection
c. Trace metals
d. Blood disorders

39. If the phlebotomist notes that an aliquot of serum contains a fibrin clot, the most likely reason is that:

a. The serum was improperly transferred from the specimen tube.
b. The specimen was stored at the incorrect temperature.
c. Centrifugation was carried out before clotting was complete.
d. The centrifuge was unbalanced.

40. The temperature of a heel-warming device used to increase blood flow in a neonate should not exceed:

a. 36 °C
b. 42 °C
c. 48 °C
d. 50 °C

41. Which of the following tests or panels is NOT part of dementia screening?

a. HIV antibody test
b. Kidney function panel
c. Thyroid function panel
d. Liver function panel

42. Following a venipuncture in the antecubital area, the arm should remain bandaged for a minimum of:

a. 5 minutes
b. 15 minutes
c. 30 minutes
d. 60 minutes

43. To obtain the peak level of an oral drug, a blood sample should usually be drawn:

    a. 30–60 minutes after the dose
    b. 1–2 hours after the dose
    c. 2–4 hours after the dose
    d. 4–6 hours after the dose

44. The laboratory test that is most affected by hemolysis is:

    a. TP
    b. Ca
    c. Acid phosphatase
    d. K

45. Waived tests are:

    a. CLIA-designated tests that are fairly simple and carry a low risk of error
    b. Tests that cannot be carried out by phlebotomists
    c. Complex tests that require special handling
    d. Tests that are not required for a specific diagnosis

46. If a patient is markedly obese, the first site to check for vein access is the:

    a. Antecubital area
    b. Lateral wrist
    c. Dorsal metacarpal veins
    d. Mid forearm

47. Which of the following items generally require only cleaning and NOT disinfection or sterilization?

    a. IV pumps
    b. Light switches
    c. Surgical instruments
    d. Bed curtains

48. When the patient begins the GTT but the FBS is 180 mg/dL, the next step is to:

    a. Notify the physician.
    b. Administer glucose solution.
    c. Administer water to drink.
    d. Discontinue testing.

49. Which of the following statements regarding arterial puncture is FALSE?

    a. Arterial puncture is more difficult to perform than venipuncture.
    b. Arterial puncture is used to evaluate ABGs.
    c. Arterial puncture is used for routine blood tests.
    d. Arterial puncture is more painful than venipuncture.

50. When attempting venipuncture on a rolling vein, the vein is likely to move:

    a. Up and down
    b. Laterally
    c. Proximally
    d. Distally

51. **If asked to transport a urine specimen to the laboratory, the phlebotomist should know that the longest the specimen can be stored at room temperature is:**
    a. 30 minutes
    b. 1 hour
    c. 1.5 hours
    d. 2 hours

52. **The most common pattern for antecubital veins is:**
    a. H-shaped
    b. B-shaped
    c. I-shaped
    d. M-shaped

53. **The primary reason that a blood test is scheduled for a predawn hour when the patient is normally sleeping is:**
    a. Diurnal variation
    b. Staff availability
    c. Error in order
    d. Patient anxiety

54. **If the antecubital veins cannot be used for specimen collection, the next site to consider is the:**
    a. Dorsal surface of the hand
    b. Palmar surface of the hand
    c. Lateral wrist, thumb side
    d. Dorsal surface of the foot

55. **Which of the following statements regarding HIV is FALSE?**
    a. HIV may be transmitted through breast milk.
    b. No vaccine is available for HIV.
    c. Postexposure treatment is recommended for all occupational exposures.
    d. Those exposed to HIV must be retested 6 months after exposure.

56. **A viral infection may result in increased:**
    a. Neutrophils
    b. Lymphocytes
    c. Monocytes
    d. Thrombocytes

57. **With the exception of the label, the AABB pink-capped evacuated collection tube is the same as the:**
    a. Green-capped
    b. Light-blue–capped
    c. Lavender-capped
    d. Red-capped

163

58. Which of the following governmental agencies requires the use of needleless blood transfer devices?

a. CMS
b. FDA
c. CDC
d. OSHA

59. Increased levels of which of the following are associated with heart attack?

a. Albumin
b. PSA
c. CK
d. CEA

60. If, when the phlebotomist arrives to do a venipuncture, the patient states that she has been calling for 20 minutes for a nurse to help her to the bathroom but no one has answered, the best initial response is to:

a. Get a nurse to assist the patient.
b. Complete the venipuncture quickly.
c. Assist the patient to the bathroom.
d. Return at a later time.

61. The initial screening test for thyroid dysfunction is usually:

a. TSH
b. T3
c. T4
d. Anti-TPO

62. Which of the following tests are NOT performed on whole blood?

a. HBV antibody
b. CBC
c. ESR
d. Hgb electrophoresis

63. When performing filter paper collection for newborn screening, the phlebotomist should NOT:

a. Air dry the filter paper.
b. Warm the heel before puncture.
c. Wipe off the first blood drop.
d. Apply >1 gtt per collection paper.

64. Which of the following activities is allowed in the laboratory?

a. Drinking fluids
b. Pipetting by mouth
c. Smelling chemicals
d. Telephoning

65. For a patient receiving warfarin (Coumadin), the INR is usually maintained at:

a. 0.5–1.0
b. 1–2
c. 2–3
d. 3–4

66. The maximum length of time a tourniquet should be left in place is:

a. 1 minute
b. 2 minutes
c. 3 minutes
d. 4 minutes

67. If the phlebotomist is unable to locate an adequate venipuncture site with a tourniquet applied, for how long should the tourniquet be released before it is reapplied?

a. 30 seconds
b. 1 minute
c. 2 minutes
d. 3 minutes

68. Which of the following substances that may be present in collection tubes is NOT an anticoagulant?

a. Sodium fluoride
b. Sodium citrate
c. ACD (acid citrate dextrose)
d. Potassium oxalate

69. In a collection tube of separated whole blood, the buffy coat is composed of:

a. WBCs and platelets
b. RBCs
c. Plasma
d. Lipids

70. If the phlebotomist must don PPE to enter an airborne isolation room, in which order should the PPE be donned (first to last)?

a. Respirator, face shield, gloves, gown
b. Face shield, gloves, gown, respirator
c. Gown, gloves, respirator, face shield
d. Gown, respirator, face shield, gloves

71. When a patient is suspected of having septicemia, what is the minimum recommended number of sets of blood cultures?

a. Two
b. Three
c. Four
d. Five

72. **Which of the following is an example of vector transmission?**
    a. Tuberculosis
    b. Salmonella infection
    c. Bubonic plague
    d. HIV

73. **Which of the following is an acceptable part of professional behavior?**
    a. Pointing out an error in collection tube selection
    b. Using the telephone during a meeting
    c. Failing to greet coworkers when entering the lab
    d. Arriving to a meeting late

74. **Which of the following is the appropriate level of isolation for a patient with influenza?**
    a. Droplet
    b. Contact
    c. Airborne
    d. Standard

75. **Which vein is recommended as the first choice for venipuncture per CLSI guidelines?**
    a. Cephalic
    b. Median cubital
    c. Basilic
    d. Brachial

76. **If blood must be drawn from an arm that has an IV in place, the IV should first be turned off for at least:**
    a. 1 minute
    b. 2 minutes
    c. 4 minutes
    d. 6 minutes

77. **Which of the following is an appropriate method of applying pressure to stop bleeding after venipuncture in the antecubital area?**
    a. Applying a gauze pressure dressing
    b. Flexing the elbow sharply
    c. Applying a cotton ball pressure dressing
    d. Maintaining direct pressure for 3–5 seconds

78. **When an infection is spread through droplets, the phlebotomist should don:**
    a. Gloves
    b. Gloves and a mask/face shield
    c. Gloves, gown, and a mask/face shield
    d. Gloves, gown, N95 respirator, and eye protection

79. **When doing a fingerstick on an adult, it is most appropriate to use the:**
    a. Thumb (1st)
    b. Middle finger (3rd)
    c. Index finger (2nd)
    d. Little finger (5th)

80. During a venipuncture, if the needle goes through the vein and a hematoma begins to rapidly develop, the next step is to:

- a. Complete the blood draw and then apply pressure.
- b. Remove the needle and tourniquet and elevate the arm.
- c. Complete the blood draw and apply an ice compress.
- d. Remove the needle and tourniquet and apply pressure.

81. Which of the following pieces of information does NOT have to be provided to patients as part of informed consent?

- a. Methods
- b. Risks
- c. Benefits
- d. Cost of testing

82. The primary reason that a young child may appear more cooperative and cry less during venipuncture when no parent is present is because without a parent, the child is likely:

- a. More afraid
- b. Less afraid
- c. Less attention seeking
- d. Less spoiled

83. Which of the following is NOT an example of a preanalytical error?

- a. Incorrect patient ID on printed lab results
- b. Blood drawn from an edematous arm
- c. Incorrect additive in specimen
- d. Tourniquet left in place for 3 minutes

84. Wearing artificial nails increases the risk of harboring:

- a. Fungi
- b. Viruses
- c. Gram-negative bacteria
- d. Gram-positive bacteria

85. When collecting a blood sample from a geriatric patient, it is important to recognize that the:

- a. Veins are more likely to collapse or roll.
- b. Veins are more difficult to identify.
- c. Blood flow is often stronger.
- d. Skin is more elastic.

86. When conducting a heelstick on an infant, the puncture depth should not exceed:

- a. 1 mm
- b. 2 mm
- c. 3 mm
- d. 4 mm

87. If the laboratory has gotten new equipment with which the phlebotomist is not familiar, the best solution is to:

    a. Request training.
    b. Refuse to use the equipment.
    c. Try to use the equipment.
    d. Ask other staff to assist.

88. For which of the following evacuated collection tubes is the minimum acceptable draw volume 100%?

    a. Light-blue–capped and yellow-capped
    b. Red-capped and lavender-capped
    c. Green-capped and gray-capped
    d. Yellow-capped and green-capped

89. According to CLSI guidelines, when using a variety of tubes, needles, and holders, the phlebotomist should first ensure that they:

    a. Have the same manufacturer
    b. Appear compatible
    c. Are in correct sizes
    d. Are intact

90. Which of the following statements regarding hCG testing is FALSE?

    a. Contaminants such as detergent may invalidate results.
    b. Medications may produce false-negative results.
    c. Positive results are available the first week after conception.
    d. Ovarian tumors may increase levels.

91. When collecting nasopharyngeal secretions with a flexible swab, the patient's head should be inclined back from 90° (vertical) to:

    a. 80°
    b. 70°
    c. 60°
    d. 50°

92. Which of the following is NOT used for coagulation monitoring?

    a. ACT
    b. Hgb
    c. PT
    d. PTT

93. When a specimen requires immediate chilling, the appropriate procedure is to:

    a. Place the specimen on cubes of ice.
    b. Place the specimen in a mixture of ice and water.
    c. Place the specimen in the refrigerator.
    d. Place the specimen on dry ice.

94. STAT blood tests are often performed on plasma rather than serum because:

a. Serum requires longer processing time.
b. Plasma provides better accuracy.
c. Plasma collection is easier.
d. Plasma tests are less expensive.

95. Prior to a 3-hour GTT, the patient should fast for at least:

a. 2 hours
b. 6 hours
c. 8 hours
d. 12 hours

96. If 3 tubes, each containing 2 mL of CSF, are collected, which tube should be used for C&S?

a. First
b. Second
c. Third
d. Order does not matter

97. The maximum volume of blood that a person can donate to a blood bank at one time is:

a. 200 mL
b. 250 mL
c. 500 mL
d. 650 mL

98. If the phlebotomist is unable to obtain a specimen when attempting a venipuncture, which of the following actions should generally be avoided?

a. Slightly withdrawing the needle
b. Slightly inserting the needle further
c. Probing laterally
d. Removing the needle and starting over

99. When drawing blood from a patient in isolation for infection with *Clostridioides difficile*, gloves should be donned:

a. After palpating the site
b. Before entering the room
c. Immediately before preparing the site
d. Immediately after preparing the site

100. Which equipment poses the greatest risk of transfer of bacteria in a hospital?

a. Floors
b. Bedside tables
c. Bed rails
d. Door handles

101. If venipuncture is attempted and no blood returns when the evacuated tube is attached but the needle appears to be in the vein, the initial response should be to:

    a. Consider an ankle vein.
    b. Remove the needle.
    c. Reposition the needle.
    d. Change the evacuated tube.

102. What is the recommended minimum time a blood specimen should be allowed to clot to produce a quality sample?

    a. 5 minutes
    b. 10 minutes
    c. 20 minutes
    d. 30 minutes

103. The _____ is a type of exocrine gland.

    a. pancreas
    b. pituitary
    c. thyroid
    d. sweat gland

104. Where should the tourniquet be placed in reference to the venipuncture site?

    a. 5–10 cm superior
    b. 5–10 cm inferior
    c. 5–10 cm posterior
    d. 5–10 cm anterior

105. Which of the following tests requires fasting for accuracy?

    a. Glucose
    b. CBC
    c. Electrolytes
    d. WBC count

106. If a physician has ordered venipuncture for blood C&S, CBC, and BMP for an adult patient, what is the correct order of draw (first to last)?

    a. C&S, CBC, BMP
    b. C&S, BMP, CBC
    c. CBC, BMP, C&S
    d. CBC, C&S, BMP

107. If, after the phlebotomist completes a venipuncture that required fasting, the patient asks for a drink of water but none is available at beside, the phlebotomist should:

    a. Get the patient a glass of water.
    b. Refer the request to a nurse.
    c. Tell the patient no water is available.
    d. Tell the patient he is not allowed water.

108. Exercise increases blood levels of all of the following EXCEPT:
a. Protein
b. Cholesterol
c. Liver enzymes
d. Skeletal muscle enzymes

109. *Accessioning of specimens* refers to:
a. Receiving and recording samples into the laboratory
b. Processing samples brought to the lab
c. Sorting laboratory samples according to the tests required
d. Documenting the results of laboratory tests

110. Troponin is used in the diagnosis of:
a. Diabetes
b. Heart attack
c. Anemia
d. Colon cancer

111. For inpatients, warning signs, such as "fall precautions," are usually placed on the:
a. Foot of the patient's bed
b. Wall behind the patient's head
c. Patient's door
d. Patient's armband

112. Which of the following procedures is NOT used to help visualize superficial veins?
a. Tapping the vein
b. Applying warm, moist compress
c. Raising the arm
d. Massaging (distal to proximal)

113. An FBS that is ordered QID a.c. and h.s. must be done:
a. 3 times daily, before meals and at bedtime
b. 3 times daily, after meals and at bedtime
c. 4 times daily, before meals and at bedtime
d. 4 times daily, after meals and at bedtime

114. How many drops of blood are required for newborn blood spot collection on a screening card?
a. 2
b. 3
c. 4
d. 5

115. The type of fluid that is collected with a thoracentesis is:
a. Peritoneal
b. Pericardial
c. Pleural
d. Synovial

116. The act of pumping the fist during venipuncture risks which of the following errors in test results?

    a. Higher level of calcium

    b. Higher level of potassium

    c. Higher level of lactate

    d. Lower level of sodium

117. The myocardial infarction panel does NOT include:

    a. Troponin I

    b. Myoglobin

    c. CK-MB

    d. Creatinine

118. Which of the following tests is NOT part of enzyme studies for a heart attack?

    a. Myoglobin

    b. Troponin

    c. CK-BB

    d. CK-MB

119. In most states, the qualifications of phlebotomists are determined by:

    a. State licensing requirements

    b. Accreditation agencies

    c. Employers

    d. CLSI

120. Which of the following is NOT usually required on a computer-generated requisition for a blood test?

    a. Patient's name and birthdate

    b. Patient allergies/sensitivities

    c. Test status (specific guidelines)

    d. Patient's address

Answer Key and Explanations for Test #3

1. C: The Americans with Disabilities Act (ADA) governs the accommodations that must be made in the laboratory for patients and workers who use wheelchairs. The 1992 ADA is civil rights legislation that provides people with disabilities, including those with mental impairment, access to employment and to the community. The ADA covers not only obvious disabilities but also disorders such as arthritis, seizure disorders, and cardiovascular and respiratory disorders.

2. D: Fires are classified according to the type of material that is burning, with an electrical fire classified as type C. Fire extinguishers are classified according to the type of fire that they extinguish, so the ABC fire extinguisher (commonly found in healthcare facilities) will extinguish type A fires (ordinary combustible materials), type B fires (flammable liquids), and type C fires (electrical). The phlebotomist should always know the locations of fire extinguishers throughout the lab and the facility and should know how to use them in an emergency.

3. B: Dwarfism can be caused by hypofunctioning of the pituitary gland in childhood; this form is known as pituitary dwarfism. Cushing syndrome is caused by hypersecretion of the glucocorticoid hormone. Type 1 diabetes is thought to be caused by an autoimmune disorder; type 2 diabetes is caused by reduced secretion of insulin from the pancreas. Parkinson's disease is a disorder of the peripheral nervous system.

4. C: Specimens for some tests should be protected from light because light may cause the substances that are to be tested to deteriorate. For example, bilirubin levels may decrease by half within an hour if exposed to light. Other blood tests that require that specimens be protected from light include vitamin A, vitamin B6, beta-carotene, and porphyrins. Capillary tubes that block light are available to protect specimens. Collection tubes may also be immediately wrapped in aluminum foil or placed in a special canister that blocks light.

5. B: If a patient continuously rubs her hands together and licks her lips when the phlebotomist is explaining a procedure, the phlebotomist should consider that the patient is likely nervous. Rubbing the hands together is a self-comforting method, and stress may reduce salivation (i.e., cause dry mouth), causing the patient to lick her lips. Paying close attention to a patient's body language may help the phlebotomist better evaluate the patient's emotional status and respond to the patient's needs.

6. B: The maximum size of syringe that should be used for blood collection is 10 mL. As the size of the syringe increases, the vacuum created when withdrawing blood also increases, so the vein may collapse if the syringe is too large, especially in older adults or those with small and/or fragile veins. If more than a 10 mL sample of blood is needed, then it is better to use a winged infusion set with a syringe attached or a needle with evacuated collection tubes.

7. B: If a specimen must be refrigerated, the temperature should be 2–10 °C (35.6–50 °F). If the specimen must be frozen, the temperature must be maintained at –20 °C (–4 °F), although some specimens require freezing to –70 °C (–94 °F) or colder, so the requirements for each type of specimen should always be verified.

8. A: According to CLSI standards, while inside the laboratory the phlebotomist should wear a long-sleeved laboratory coat/gown that is closed in the front. These garments should not be worn outside of the laboratory. They may be made of disposable material. Any open area, such as a cut or puncture, should be covered with an impermeable dressing to prevent contact with blood or other body fluids. The phlebotomist should wear gloves in areas set up to receive specimens.

9. C: The Allen test is used to assess collateral circulation. In performing the Allen test, both the radial and ulnar arteries should be compressed at the same time to assess the return of blood when pressure is released. The patient should not hyperextend the fingers when opening his or her hand because this may result in decreased blood flow and interfere with results. A positive result is indicated when the hand flushes pink or returns to normal color within 15 seconds.

10. B: According to the order of the draw for venous blood, blood cultures are always drawn first to ensure that there is no contamination. The order of the draw is as follows:

1. Blood cultures
2. Light blue (sodium citrate)
3. Red, red speckled, gold (clot activators, gels)
4. Light green, dark green, speckled green (heparin, with or without gel separator)
5. Lavender/purple, pearl, pink (EDTA, with or without gel separator)
6. Gray (sodium fluoride/potassium oxalate glycolytic inhibitor)

11. A: With outpatients, urine specimens should be collected prior to venipuncture because patients may feel light-headed and faint in the bathroom after venipuncture, increasing the risk of injury. If the patient has locked the door or there is no obvious indication that the patient has fainted, the patient may not receive needed first aid for an extended time. Generally, venipuncture should be the last test carried out when tests of multiple body fluids are ordered.

12. A: Immunologic tests use antibodies and antigens to detect a response to disease; immunologic tests include HIV (human immunodeficiency virus) and HBV (hepatitis B virus). Coagulation tests use the clotting mechanisms of the blood for both diagnostic purposes and to monitor anticoagulation therapy; these tests include PT (prothrombin time), aPTT (activated partial thromboplastin time), INR (international normalized ratio), and fibrinogen level. Microbiologic tests use blood samples to identify pathogenic agents; these tests include a wide range of C&S (cultures and sensitivities). Chemical testing measures amounts of biochemical factors in blood; these tests include BMP (basic metabolic panel), CMP (comprehensive metabolic panel), and FBS (fasting blood sugar).

13. B: Phlebotomists are most likely to develop sensitivity to latex because of wearing latex gloves. Exposure to other sources of latex, such as in tourniquets, latex-capped collection tubes, and medical equipment (e.g., blood pressure cuffs, stethoscopes) may exacerbate sensitivity. Contact dermatitis with itching and redness is the most common symptom, but some people may develop severe anaphylaxis.

14. A: Albumin is included in a hepatic (liver) function panel. A hepatic function panel evaluates the liver functions, which include producing proteins, producing and storing lipids, metabolizing and storing carbohydrates, producing and secreting bile, and metabolizing and secreting bilirubin and toxins. Liver function may be impaired by infection, inflammation, trauma, tumors, and toxins. Tests included in a hepatic function panel include alanine transaminase (ALT), albumin, albumin/globulin ratio, alkaline phosphatase (ALP), aspartate aminotransferase (AST), direct bilirubin, globulin, total bilirubin, and total protein.

15. B: When collecting blood specimens with collection tubes, the beginning of the correct order of draw (first to last) is (1) yellow tops, (2) light blue tops, and (3) red tops, per CLSI recommendations. The order of draw must be carefully adhered to because the transfer needle may

174

become contaminated with additives, and this contamination may affect the outcomes of tests. Blood cultures are always collected first to minimize the risk of bacterial contamination.

16. C: According to the American Hospital Association's *The Patient Care Partnership,* patients do NOT have the right to expect cost-effective care. Patient rights include:

- High-quality care: includes knowing the names and qualifications of caregivers
- Clean and safe environment: includes freedom from errors, abuse, and neglect
- Privacy protection: includes being provided with notice of privacy practices and adherence to regulations regarding privacy, such as HIPAA (Health Insurance Portability and Accountability Act)
- Involvement in care: includes discussions of medical condition(s), treatment options, treatment plan, and decision making
- Discharge planning: includes identifying community resources and coordination of care
- Assistance with billing claims: includes filing claims

17. D: Because type O blood lacks antigens, an individual with type O blood can be a donor to individuals with any of the four blood types; thus, a person with type O blood is known as a universal donor.

18. A: The organization that develops and publishes the National Patient Safety Goals (NPSGs) is The Joint Commission, which is an accrediting agency for various types of medical facilities, including laboratories, critical access hospitals, behavioral health facilities, and ambulatory health facilities. NPSGs are published yearly. NPSGs for laboratories in 2025 include identifying patients correctly with 2 identifiers, improving staff communication by ensuring test results get to the correct person in a timely manner, and preventing infection by following CDC hand cleaning guidelines.

19. A: If doing a venipuncture on a patient with small, fragile veins, the best solution is to use a winged infusion set with a syringe rather than an evacuated tube, because small veins tend to collapse easily when using an evacuated tube. The syringe allows the phlebotomist to gently withdraw the blood. A winged infusion set has a smaller and shorter needle and is less likely to go through the vein during the venipuncture.

20. B: When entering a room to draw blood from an individual on contact precautions, the PPE (personal protective equipment) that is generally required is gown and gloves. The gown should be applied before the gloves, and both removed at the door upon leaving the room. Additional PPE is needed only if the person entering the room is likely to encounter spray or splashes of body fluids, such when a wound is being irrigated or a patient suctioned of oral secretions.

21. C: Most microcollection tubes that contain anticoagulants require 8–10 inversions after the addition of blood to ensure that the additive and blood are mixed adequately. Microcollection tubes with anticoagulants that require 8–10 inversions include:

- Lavender: K_2EDTA
- Green: lithium heparin
- Light green: lithium heparin with gel plasma separator

Gold-capped tubes contain a clot activator and gel plasma separator and require 5–10 inversions, while blue-capped tubes containing sodium citrate (an anticoagulant) require 3–4 inversions.

22. B: If a hospital laboratory is accredited by CAP (College of American Pathologists), the accreditation is reviewed every 2 years by teams of inspectors. Laboratories must meet rigorous standards as outlined by checklists. If a laboratory is accredited by CAP, CMS (Centers for Medicare and Medicaid Services) does not require further inspection. The Joint Commission also recognizes CAP accreditation. CAP accreditation usually requires higher standards than regulatory agencies because its goal is to promote the highest laboratory quality and patient safety.

23. B: The outermost layer of the skin is known as the epidermis. The second layer, or the dermis, is thicker than the epidermis and is known as the "true skin." The subcutaneous layer, or hypodermis, lies underneath the dermis.

24. B: Because both overfilling and underfilling may result in inaccurate test results or clotting, the phlebotomist should redraw blood for both tubes. Blood can never be withdrawn from one collection tube and inserted into another, even if both tubes contain the same type of additive, because this process will alter the additive to blood ratio. The phlebotomist should wait until the blood stops filling the tube by the preset vacuum volume in order to prevent underfilling and should note the line on the tube to prevent overfilling.

25. C: If the laboratory institutes policy and procedural changes, the phlebotomist should expect to receive appropriate training. If training is not already planned, the phlebotomist should ask for training, explaining the reasons why the training is needed. Approaches to training may vary widely, depending on the type and extent of changes being instituted. Without training, new policies and procedures are often adopted piecemeal and without consistency, increasing risks to staff and patients as well as liability risks.

26. B: There is postexposure prophylaxis available and recommended for many diseases, including influenza, measles, pertussis, meningococcal meningitis, chickenpox, hepatitis A, HIV, and rabies. Postexposure prophylaxis for measles, chickenpox, hepatitis A, and rabies includes vaccination, whereas postexposure prophylaxis for influenza, pertussis, meningococcal meningitis, and HIV consists of antimicrobials.

27. B: The C-hold (anchoring the vein with the index finger above the venipuncture site and the thumb below) increases the risk of needlestick because the index finger is above the needle; when the needle is inserted and withdrawn (or if the patient jerks and the needle accidentally comes out), the needle may easily stick the finger. If necessary (such as with rolling veins), the vein can be anchored with a finger across the vein below the venipuncture site.

28. B: Gout is a form of arthritis affecting the joints of the feet. It is caused by increased uric acid levels in the blood. Bursitis is an inflammation of the bursa (a fluid-filled sac) between a bone and the softer tissues, such as muscles and tendons, that surround it. Rickets is a condition in children caused by lack of vitamin D and is marked by softening and malformation of the bones. A slipped disc is a condition in which the disc between two vertebrae of the spine ruptures or protrudes out of place.

29. B: The cap color for the collection tube used for tests of therapeutic drug levels is green. The green-capped collection tubes are coated on the inside with lithium heparin or sodium heparin for anticoagulation. Green-topped collection tubes are used for most chemistry tests when the tests are performed on plasma. These collection tubes should not be utilized for lithium testing if the tubes contain lithium heparin and should not be used for sodium testing if the tubes contain sodium heparin.

30. B: The veins that should not be used for venipuncture are those on the palmar side of the hand because they tend to be very small and the arteries and nerves lie in close proximity to the veins, increasing the risk of nerve damage. According to standards produced by the Clinical and Laboratory Standards Institute (CLSI), the palmar side should not be used. While not all laboratories choose to participate in CLSI, most follow the good practice standards that CLSI has established.

31. B: The proper use of a disinfectant is on inanimate objects, such as environmental surfaces and non-critical equipment, such as blood pressure cuffs. Disinfection differs from sterilization in that disinfection reduces the number of microorganisms but does not kill all of them. Sterilization is performed when all microorganisms and spores are destroyed. Sterilization is essential for critical items, which can readily spread infection because they contact sterile tissue and/or the vascular system. Critical items include venipuncture needles and IV catheters.

32. C: If a patient complains of feeling faint during collection of a blood specimen, the tourniquet and needle should be removed; pressure applied; and then the patient reclined, lain flat, or have his or her head and arms lowered. Tight clothing, especially around the neck and chest, should be loosened. Ammonia inhalants are no longer used because their use may result in adverse effects. Personnel trained in first aid should be notified so they can examine and monitor the patient.

33. C: After a blood specimen is collected in a tube that contains EDTA, the tube should be inverted 8–10 times per CLSI recommendations. Inverting the tube consists of slowly rotating the tube until the stopper is on the bottom and then back to upright to mix the sample with the additive. Shaking the tube must be avoided. Different additives require different numbers of inversions. Tubes with sodium citrate should be inverted 3–4 times, while those with a clot activator should be inverted 5–10 times. Tubes containing sodium or lithium heparin or sodium fluoride should be inverted 5–10 times.

34. B: Chemical hazards include preservatives used in the laboratory as well as all other chemicals, such as acids, that may result in burns or injury. Biologic hazards include pathogenic agents, such as viruses, bacteria, fungi, and parasites, which may be transmitted from blood and other specimens. Physical hazards include wet floors (which can cause falls), heavy objects (which may result in back injuries if lifted incorrectly), and inappropriately stored items (which may fall or block passages). Fire/explosive hazards include oxygen and combustible materials or chemicals. Sharps hazards include needles, lancets, syringes, and broken glass.

35. C: Occasionally, the name of the ordering physician, room number, or bed number on the patient's ID band may differ from these details on the requisition form. Patient identity must always be verified before collecting blood. As part of informed consent, patients have the right to refuse any blood draw (with a few legal exceptions such as court-ordered drug testing); thus, the phlebotomist must ask the patient's permission before collecting blood.

36. D: Shoulder-length or longer hair is acceptable in the laboratory if it is tied back. Wearing nail polish or large or dangling earrings is not acceptable. A laboratory coat should never be worn when leaving the lab for any reason.

37. C: Evacuated collection tubes can be stored at 4–25 °C (39.2–77 °F). Storage at temperatures outside this range may affect the integrity of the tube. Expiration dates are stamped on the tubes and should always be checked prior to use because the reliability of the vacuum and additive cannot be guaranteed beyond that time. Care should be exercised to ensure that tubes are not dropped or jostled unnecessarily. Most evacuated collection tubes are now made of plastic for safety reasons.

38. B: The C-urea breath test is used to detect the presence of *Helicobacter pylori*, a form of bacteria that causes chronic gastritis, which can eventually lead to peptic ulcer. The hydrogen breath test is used to assess lactose intolerance. Bone marrow biopsy is used to test for blood disorders. Hair samples, fingernails, blood, and urine can all be used to detect trace or heavy metals.

39. C: If the phlebotomist notes than an aliquot of serum contains a fibrin clot, the most likely reason is that centrifugation was carried out before clotting was complete. Fibrin clots are likely to form if hemolysis occurs, usually from mishandling a specimen or leaving the tourniquet on for too long. Fibrin clots may appear as globules (opaque or gelatinous) or strands in serum or plasma. In most cases, an aliquot with a fibrin clot needs to be discarded.

40. B: The temperature of a heel-warming device used to increase blood flow in a neonate should not exceed 42 °C (107.6 °F). Warming devices are especially useful for heelsticks because they can increase the flow of blood by up to 7 times, but great care must be used to avoid burning the infant. While a wet warm cloth may be applied to increase circulation, a commercial heel-warming device is safer and more effective because it maintains a stable temperature.

41. D: Liver function tests are not part of dementia screening, which is done to try to differentiate Alzheimer's disease from dementia related to other disorders. Dementia screening includes general tests for disorders that may present with dementia as one of the symptoms. Tests include thyroid and kidney function tests as well as WBC (white blood cell count) and RBC (red blood cell count). Other tests include HIV antibody, vitamin B12, syphilis screening, ESR (erythrocyte sedimentation rate), alanine transaminase, aluminum, and toxicology screening.

42. B: Per CLSI guidelines, following venipuncture in the antecubital area, the arm should remain bandaged for a minimum of 15 minutes and up to 60 minutes. Pressure should be applied with a gauze pad for 3–5 minutes and then the site checked to ensure that bleeding has stopped. If bleeding persists for more than 5 minutes, this may indicate a clotting problem and must be reported to a nurse or supervisor immediately. Patients should not be asked to flex the arm to apply pressure on the vein.

43. B: To obtain the peak level of an oral drug, a blood sample should usually be drawn 1 to 2 hours after a dose. If the medication was administered IM, then the peak level is usually taken 1 hour after a dose; and if IV, 30 minutes. However, physicians may specify a different time depending on the information provided by manufacturers regarding peak levels. In all cases, the phlebotomist should verify that the medication was actually administered at the scheduled time prior to collecting the blood sample.

44. D: Of the laboratory tests listed, the test that is most affected by hemolysis is K (potassium). Other tests that are equally affected include LH (lactate dehydrogenase), AST (aspartate aminotransferase), and the CBC (complete blood count). Fe (serum iron), ALT (alanine aminotransferase, and T4 (thyroxine) are also noticeably affected. Tests that are only mildly affected include P (phosphorous), TP (total protein), albumin, Mg (magnesium), Ca (calcium), and acid phosphatase.

45. A: Waived tests are Clinical Laboratory Improvement Amendments (CLIA)-designated tests that are fairly simple and carry a low risk of error, so they are generally reliable if carried out properly and if the equipment is in operating condition. Most point-of-care (POC) tests are waived, although not all are. Phlebotomists may only carry out POC tests that are waived. Waived POC tests may be used in the home environment. For example, glucometers are used by both healthcare providers and patients to monitor blood sugar.

46. A: If a patient is markedly obese, the first site to check is the antecubital area because patients often exhibit a double crease in that area, and the median cubital vein can often be easily palpated and accessed within that creased space. If the phlebotomist is unable to locate the median cubital vein, the cephalic vein may sometimes be accessed if the arm is rotated medially. The phlebotomist may also ask the patient where blood draws have been successful previously.

47. D: The item that generally requires only cleaning and not disinfection or sterilization is bed curtains. Cleaning involves removing debris (such as dirt, dust, and food) in non-critical items, such as walls, windows, and floors, although in some cases cleaning is followed by disinfection according to protocols established by the facility. Other items that are usually only cleaned include furniture in waiting areas (used by clothed individuals) and rooms in non-patient care areas, such as administrative offices.

48. A: When the patient begins the GTT (glucose tolerance test) but the FBS (fasting blood sugar) is 180 mg/dL, the next step is to notify the physician because drinking oral glucose with an elevated FBS may put the patient at risk of severe hyperglycemia. The GTT measures glucose levels at preset intervals to determine if patients are able to adequately metabolize glucose at a normal rate; failure to do so may be an indication of diabetes, hyperthyroidism, or alcoholic liver disease.

49. C: Arterial puncture is primarily performed to evaluate arterial blood gasses (ABGs). Arterial puncture is usually more difficult to perform and is more painful than venipuncture; thus, it is not used for routine blood tests.

50. B: When attempting venipuncture on a rolling vein, the vein is likely to move laterally because it is not firmly attached to the tissue. Rolling veins are most common in infants and older adults, but they are not uncommon and can occur in any patient. Veins are more likely to roll if the needle punctures the vein on the side rather than in the middle. Stretching the skin tautly and anchoring the vein well with the thumb can help to prevent the vein from rolling.

51. D: If asked to transport a urine specimen to the laboratory, the phlebotomist should know that the longest the specimen can be stored at room temperature is 2 hours. If a urine specimen will not be processed within 60 minutes, it may be transferred into a urinalysis tube that contains a preservative. If the specimen is unpreserved and processing will be delayed beyond 2 hours, the specimen must be protected from exposure to light and can be refrigerated for up to 24 hours.

52. A: The most common pattern for antecubital veins is H-shaped, which occurs in about 70% of the population, with the remaining people primarily exhibiting the M-shape. With the H-shape pattern, the most accessible vein is the median cubital, which crosses near the center of the antecubital area and is more superficial than other vessels. With the M-shaped pattern, the first choice for venipuncture is usually the median vein because it does not lie in close proximity to nerves or arteries.

53. A: The primary reason that a blood test is scheduled for a predawn hour when the patient is normally sleeping is diurnal variation. Diurnal variation refers to normal variations that occur at different times in the 24-hour circadian cycle. Tests that may be ordered in the very early morning hours include renin and TSH (thyroid-stimulating hormone) levels. Other tests that have peak levels in the morning include bilirubin, insulin, iron, K (potassium), RBCs, and testosterone. In contrast, the following tests show lowest levels in the morning: creatinine, glucose, triglycerides, eosinophils, and phosphate.

54. A: If the antecubital veins cannot be used for specimen collection, the next site to consider is the dorsal (top) surface of the hand. The veins on the lateral wrist above the thumb lie near the radial nerve, so this site should be avoided. The palmar surface of the hand poses increased risk of nerve and tendon involvement. The veins in the foot should not be used without specific physician orders because of an increased risk of necrosis and thrombophlebitis.

55. C: Because exposure does not necessarily lead to human immunodeficiency virus (HIV), as well as the potential for serious drug side effects, postexposure treatment is not recommended for most occupational exposures to HIV. No vaccine is available for HIV, and HIV may be transmitted through breast milk. Those exposed to HIV should be tested 6 weeks, 12 weeks, and 6 months after exposure.

56. B: A viral infection may result in increased lymphocytes, which are one type of white blood cell (WBC). Lymphocytes usually comprise 24–44% of the total WBCs in adults. A bacterial infection often results in decreased lymphocytes but increased neutrophils. Increased lymphocyte count is also commonly found with some diseases, so it is not specific to viral infections. Conditions associated with increased lymphocyte count include Addison's disease, lymphocytic leukemia, ulcerative colitis, lymphomas, and lymphosarcoma.

57. C: With the exception of the label, the AABB (American Association of Blood Banks) pink-capped evacuated collection tube is the same as the lavender-capped collection tube. The pink-capped tube contains spray-dried K_2EDTA anticoagulant. The label for the pink-capped tube meets the AABB requirements for patient identification and cross-match information. The pink-capped tube is used for all blood bank testing.

58. D: OSHA requires the use of needleless blood transfer devices as a means of decreasing the risk of needlestick injuries and infection. This requirement is part of OSHA's Bloodborne Pathogen Standard. Blood transfer devices should not be reused because of the increased risks involved in removing the needle and the risk of possible contamination by blood. Sharps used for blood draw should have sharps injury protection devices whenever possible. Needles without this protection should never be recapped, as this increases risk of a needlestick.

59. C: Increased levels of creatine kinase (CK) are associated with heart attack. The PSA, or prostate specific antigen, level is used to test for prostate cancer. Carcinoembryonic antigen (CEA) is used in digestive system testing. Albumin is used in urinary system testing.

60. A: If, when the phlebotomist arrives to do a venipuncture, the patient states that she has been calling for 20 minutes for a nurse to help her to the bathroom but no one has answered, the best initial response is to get a nurse to assist the patient. The phlebotomist should not assist the patient because this may pose issues of liability. The phlebotomist may wait until the patient returns from the bathroom or return at a later time, depending on the length of time the patient needs and the phlebotomist's schedule of draws.

61. A: The initial screening test for thyroid dysfunction is usually TSH (thyroid stimulating hormone, normal range 0.4–4.2 mIU/L) because the pituitary gland releases TSH in response to levels of T3 (thyroxine) and T4 (triiodothyronine). If levels of T3 and T4 are decreased (hypothyroidism), the TSH levels will be increased. If T3 and T4 levels are increased (hyperthyroidism), the TSH levels will be decreased. Anti-TPO (anti-thyroperoxidase antibodies) is tested if thyroid dysfunction is believed to be due to an immune response.

62. A: The test that should not be performed on whole blood is the HBV antibody, which must be done on serum. Tests that must be performed only with whole blood include CBC (complete blood count), ESR (erythrocyte sedimentation rate), and hemoglobin electrophoresis (although protein electrophoresis must be done with serum). When whole blood is needed for testing, it must be collected in a tube that contains an anticoagulant to prevent clotting so the sample can be mixed well before processing.

63. D: When performing filter paper collection for newborn screening, the phlebotomist should not apply more than 1 gtt per collection paper. The first drop is wiped off, and only gentle pressure should be used to encourage further blood. After a large drop of blood collects, the filter paper is carefully touched to the blood drop (but not the skin) on one side of the collection paper only. After collection, the filter paper must be air dried for a minimum of three hours at room temperature.

64. D: Telephoning, such as to report a test result, is allowed in the laboratory, although personal calls should not be made during working hours. Drinking and eating are prohibited in the lab. Other prohibitions include handling contact lenses, storing food for human consumption, pipetting by mouth, and smoking. Mechanical pipettes must be used because of the risk of ingesting substances when pipetting by mouth. Chemicals should never be tasted or smelled because of the risk of toxicity.

65. C: For a patient receiving warfarin (Coumadin), the INR (international normalized ratio) is usually maintained at 2–3. The INR is a standardized test of the PT (prothrombin time). Warfarin is an oral anticoagulant taken to prevent blood clots. At this INR level, patients are prone to bruising and bleed easily, so hematomas may form when blood is withdrawn. Patients are often instructed in self-testing and do so at home on a weekly basis. If testing is done in a lab, it may be done on a weekly, biweekly, or even monthly basis.

66. A: The maximum length of time a tourniquet should be left in place is 1 minute, per Clinical and Laboratory Standards Institute (CLSI) recommendations. The tourniquet is usually released as soon as blood begins to flow into the evacuated tube; however, if several tubes of blood must be collected, the tourniquet is usually left in place until blood begins flowing into the last evacuated tube. Leaving the tourniquet in place for an extended period may alter the results of protein-based components and packed red cell volume.

67. C: Per Clinical and Laboratory Standards Institute (CLSI) guidelines, if the phlebotomist is unable to locate an adequate venipuncture site with a tourniquet applied, the tourniquet should be released for 2 minutes before it is reapplied in order to prevent trauma to the area and to allow blood flow to normalize. Applying the tourniquet repeatedly to the same site should also be avoided. If two or three attempts to find an adequate vein are unsuccessful, then an alternate site, such as the other arm, should be tried.

68. A: Sodium fluoride is not an anticoagulant; it is an additive used to stabilize the level of glucose in a blood specimen. Other additives include thrombin, which promotes blood clotting, and gel, which serves as a barrier between serum and cells. Anticoagulants, used to prevent the blood from clotting in collection tubes, include sodium citrate, potassium oxalate, sodium heparin, lithium heparin, K_2EDTA (potassium EDTA), Na_2EDTA (sodium EDTA), ACD (acid citrate dextrose), SPS (sodium polyanethol sulfonate), and CTAD (citrate, theophylline, adenosine, dipyridamole).

69. A: In a collection tube of separated whole blood, the buffy coat is comprised of white blood cells (WBCs) and platelets. After centrifugation of a blood specimen, three distinct layers are evident in the collection tube. The top layer (which comprises about 55%) is the plasma and the bottom layer (which comprises about 45%) is the red blood cells (RBCs). These two layers are separated by a (less than 1%) thin buff-colored layer of cells, the WBCs, and the platelets.

70. D: If the phlebotomist must don PPE to enter an airborne isolation room, the order in which the PPE should be donned is:

1. Gown
2. Respirator
3. Face shield or goggles
4. Gloves

The gown is put on first because the phlebotomist must reach around to fasten it and may contact the hair or clothes in doing so. Then, the respirator is applied, followed by the face shield, which covers the respirator. Gloves are donned last because most contact with the patients is with the hands.

71. B: When a patient is suspected of having septicemia, the minimum recommended number of sets of blood cultures is three (six total bottles) because this provides the highest chance (95–99% per CLSI evidence) of identifying the causative agent. Each draw should include a collection tube for aerobic bacteria and another for anaerobic. Each collection tube should contain 8–10 mL for adults or 0.5–5.0 mL (depending on age and weight) for children. Careful disinfection of the skin must be done prior to venipuncture to avoid contaminating the specimen with skin bacteria.

72. C: The transmission of bubonic plague by fleas from rodents is an example of vector transmission. Tuberculosis is spread via airborne transmission. Transmission of salmonella though handling contaminated food and transmission of human immunodeficiency virus (HIV) infection via a blood transfusion are examples of vehicle transmission.

73. A: Pointing out an error in collection tube selection is an acceptable part of professional behavior and shows concern for the patient and the person making the error. Errors should never be overlooked. Behaviors that are not professional include using the telephone during a meeting (except in emergency situations), failing to greet coworkers or acknowledge them in some way when entering the lab, and arriving late to a meeting because this inconveniences others.

74. A: The appropriate level of isolation for a patient with influenza is droplet precautions because the infection may be spread through droplets generated by coughing. Infections for which droplet isolation are appropriate include parainfluenza virus, RSV, *Bordetella pertussis* infection, and human metapneumovirus. Patients being treated for *Neisseria meningitides* or group A *Streptococcus* are maintained on droplet precautions for the first 24 hours of treatment. PPE includes a face mask; gloves, gown, and goggles or face shield may also be indicated.

75. B: CLSI guidelines recommend using veins located in the antecubital fossa as the preferred site for venipuncture, followed by veins on the dorsal aspect of the hand. The antecubital fossa has three major veins that may be used. Per CLSI guidelines, the order of preference starts with the median (middle) cubital vein, followed by the lateral cubital (cephalic) vein, then the medial cubital (basilic) vein. The median cubital joins the cephalic and basilic veins and is easily accessed in the antecubital space of the arm. The basilic vein lies close to the median nerve and should be the last choice for venipuncture. Additionally, the proximal portion of the vein lies near arteries. The dorsal metacarpal veins in the hands can also be used for venipuncture.

76. B: If blood must be drawn from an arm that has an IV in place, the IV should be turned off for at least 2 minutes before the specimen is collected, which allows the IV fluid to enter the circulation and reduce the dilution of the blood sample. The phlebotomist should not turn the IV off. Rather, the patient's healthcare provider (generally a nurse) must be responsible for confirming that the IV fluid is safe to turn off, turning the IV off, and then turning the IV back on upon completion of the blood collection. The phlebotomist must notify the nurse upon completion of blood collection so that the IV can be resumed as quickly as possible. It is preferable to do the venipuncture distal to the IV insertion site when possible, with the tourniquet also applied distal to the IV insertion site. The site (proximal or distal) in relation to the IV should be documented.

77. A: Applying a gauze pressure dressing is an appropriate method of applying pressure to stop bleeding after venipuncture in the antecubital area. The patient should be advised to keep the dressing in place for at least 15 minutes. Direct pressure may be applied for a few minutes by the patient (if monitored) or by the phlebotomist. Cotton and rayon balls should not be used to apply pressure to the venipuncture site because they may stick to the wound and dislodge the platelet plug.

78. C: Infections that are spread via droplets can travel long distances in the air before dropping to the ground, especially when spread through sneezing and coughing. CDC guidelines recommend that a mask and face shield be donned by all healthcare providers when entering a the room of a patient that is on droplet precautions (for instance, in cases of seasonal influenza or pertussis). When the healthcare provider is at risk for exposure to bodily fluids, such as in the case of phlebotomy practices, gloves and gown are also recommended. N95 respirators are recommended for airborne diseases (e.g., COVID-19, tuberculosis).

79. B: When doing a finger stick on an adult or child over one year, it is most appropriate to use the middle finger (3rd) or the ring finger (4th) with punctures on the palmar side only and made perpendicular to the fingerprint ridges, rather than parallel to them. This recommendation is agreed upon by both CLSI and the CDC. The puncture should be made slightly laterally, as the medial aspect and tip of the fingertip are most sensitive. Punctures should be made on the non-dominant hand when possible. The thumb, index finger (2nd), and little finger (5th) should be avoided. CLSI states that the little finger is contraindicated due to the small amount of tissue and potential for hitting bone during the puncture. The thumb is not recommended due to the risk of arterial puncture and possibility of contamination. The index finger is a heavily relied-upon finger, therefore should be avoided when possible out of convenience to the patient in addition to posing a risk for contamination.

80. D: During a venipuncture, if the needle goes through the vein and a hematoma begins to rapidly develop, the next step is to remove the needle and tourniquet, then apply pressure to prevent further loss of blood into the tissue. A hematoma may also form if the needle only partially penetrates the vessel wall, allowing blood to leak into the tissue. If blood flow stops and a small hematoma begins to form, the needle's bevel may be up against a vessel wall, so rotating it slightly may stop the leak and allow blood to flow into the collection tube.

81. D: The information that does not have to be provided to patients as part of informed consent is the cost of testing; however, if the cost is extremely high, patients should be made aware of this, especially if they lack insurance. Patients do need to be aware of the methods used to conduct the test, the risks of the test, and the benefits. If alternate methods of testing are available, patients should also be apprised of these so that they have the option to choose.

82. A: The primary reason that a young child may appear more cooperative and may cry less during venipuncture when no parent is present is because without a parent, the child is likely more afraid. While it can be distressing to deal with an uncooperative and crying child, most children are very frightened of needles and express this fear through crying. It is healthier to express feelings than to suppress them as children may do if they have no parent to comfort them.

83. A: An incorrect patient ID on a printed lab result is an example of a postanalytical error because it occurred after the testing was completed. Preanalytical errors occur prior to testing and may include a wide range of physiological factors that may affect testing, including exercise, diurnal variations, diet, age, drugs, environment, altitude, position, gender, pregnancy, and stress. Venipuncture factors include both patient's condition (e.g., burns, mastectomy, IV fluids) and technical errors, such as blood drawn from an edematous arm or a tourniquet left in place for 3 minutes.

84. C: Wearing artificial nails increases the risk of harboring gram-negative bacteria on the fingertips and may result in outbreaks of infection. The CDC recommends that artificial nails or long natural nails (which pose similar risks) should be avoided by healthcare workers who have direct contact with patients, especially in high-risk areas such as the ICU or NICU. The CDC recommends that natural nails be maintained at no longer than one-quarter inch. While unchipped nail polish poses no increased risk, chipped nail polish may harbor bacteria.

85. A: When collecting a blood sample from a geriatric patient, it is important to recognize that the veins are more likely to collapse or roll because the tissue and veins are less elastic and the veins are less secured. Older adults often have skin that is thinner and more friable, with less underlying subcutaneous fat, than that of younger people. Although this may make vessels easier to visualize, they may be more difficult to access. Blood flow may be slower because of the narrowing of vessels that occurs with age.

86. B: According to CLSI recommendations, the puncture depth of a heelstick on an infant should not exceed 2 mm because deeper punctures may result in infection or damage to the underlying bone. Heelsticks should be done only on the lateral sides of the heel and not in the central (arch) area, the posterior curve of the heel, or other parts of the foot or toes. Fingers cannot be used to obtain capillary blood in infants younger than one year.

87. A: If the laboratory has gotten new equipment with which the phlebotomist is not familiar, the best solution is to request training. Training may include one-on-one instruction by a fellow staff person, written literature, or interactive web-based training, depending on the type of equipment. The phlebotomist should not expect other staff members to assist indefinitely and should not attempt to use the equipment by trial and error. Refusing to use equipment may jeopardize employment.

88. A: The minimal acceptable draw volume is 100% of tube capacity for the light-blue–capped evacuated collection tube, which is used for coagulation tests; and the yellow-capped tube, which is used for blood cultures. For the light-blue–capped tube, overfilling can result in coagulation of the specimen and underfilling can cause prolongation of clotting times. For the yellow-capped tube, overfilling may result in clotting and underfilling can result in too small a volume of blood necessary to recover pathogenic agents.

89. A: According to CLSI guidelines, when using a variety of tubes, needles, and holders, the phlebotomist should first ensure that they have the same manufacturer. Even though equipment may appear compatible or sizes universal, there may be small differences that increase the risk of hemolysis, improper filling, or disengagement. Therefore, tubes, needles, and holders made by different manufacturers should never be combined for use. If the facility is switching to a new provider, there should be no attempt to "use up" old supplies by combining them with new items.

90. C: Human chorionic gonadotropin (hCG) levels are increased during pregnancy; however, hCG may not be present in sufficient levels for the first 2 weeks after conception, and thus may yield false-negative results on a pregnancy test. Contaminants such as detergents, protein, hematuria, and bacteria, as well as certain medications, may invalidate results. Malignant ovarian tumors and other conditions may increase hCG levels.

91. B: When collecting nasopharyngeal secretions with a flexible swab, the patient's head should be inclined from vertical (90°) to 70°. Care should be taken to not hyperextend the neck; some patients, especially older adults, may have difficulty with any extension. The swab is inserted into one nostril until it reaches the nasopharynx (at the back and top of the throat). Then, the swab is rotated a few times, gently withdrawn, and placed in a sterile container that contains transport medium.

92. B: Activated coagulation time (ACT), prothrombin time (PT), and partial thromboplastin time (PTT) are all used for coagulation monitoring. Hgb, or hemoglobin, is used for the diagnosis of anemia.

93. B: Some specimens, such as those intended for a lactate test, require immediate chilling to maintain the integrity of the sample. CLSI guidelines recommend placing the specimen immediately in a mixture of ice and water, which allows maximum contact between the cooling source and the sample tube. Large cubes of ice will not allow the maximum contact required to maintain appropriate chilling. Dry ice is not recommended due to its excessively low temperature. Refrigerating the sample is not sufficient nor does it allow chilling to continue during transport.

94. A: STAT (immediate) blood tests are often performed on plasma rather than serum because serum requires longer processing times—approximately 30 minutes for a clot to form and 10 minutes for centrifugation. Plasma can be processed immediately because it is collected in a tube with an anticoagulant, so no clot forms. The primary difference between plasma and serum is that plasma contains fibrinogen and serum does not, and the presence or absence of fibrinogen may alter some test results.

95. C: Prior to a 3-hour GTT (glucose tolerance test), the patient should fast for at least 8 hours, eating nothing and drinking only clear water. The patient should eat normal, well-balanced meals, including carbohydrates, for three days before the test. The procedure begins with a FBS (fasting blood sugar). If the FBS is within acceptable values, the patient should drink the glucose solution within 5 minutes. Blood specimens are then obtained at set times, usually at 1 hour, 2 hours, and 3 hours. The patient may eat nothing and only drink clear water until the test is completed.

96. B: If 3 tubes, each containing 2 mL of CSF (cerebrospinal fluid) are collected, the collection tube that should be used for C&S is the second tube. The specimen in the first tube is used for chemistry and immunological testing but may be contaminated with bacteria found on the skin, so it is not appropriate for C&S. The specimen in the second tube should not be contaminated with skin bacteria. The specimen in the third tube is used for cellular examination.

97. C: The maximum volume of blood that a person can donate to a blood bank at one donation is 500 mL. Requirements for blood donors include:

- Age 17 or older (16 in some states with parental permission)
- Weight: 110 lb or more; for donors 18 years and younger, minimum weight depends on height but is always at least 110 lb

Donors should bring a list of medications to ensure that they do not preclude donation of blood. Medications that may preclude donation include isotretinoin (Accutane), methotrexate, anticoagulants, and antibiotics such as metronidazole (Flagyl). In some cases, a specific period of time must elapse after discontinuing a drug before blood donation.

98. C: If the phlebotomist is unable to obtain a specimen when attempting a venipuncture, probing laterally should generally be avoided. It is painful and often unsuccessful and should only be attempted when the location of the vein has been established. If the vein is in the medial aspect of the antecubital fossa, then lateral probing should never be used because of the risk of hitting the brachial artery or a nerve. In some cases, the needle may need to be removed and an attempt made at a different site.

99. B: When drawing blood from a patient in isolation for infection with *Clostridioides difficile,* gloves should be donned before entering the room and should be kept in place throughout the procedure. This procedure should be followed for all patients in isolation. Prior to entering the room, the phlebotomist should note the type of isolation and follow standard protocols. This may include donning other PPE (personal protective equipment), such as a gown and mask and/or face shield.

100. C: The equipment that poses the greatest risk of transfer of bacteria in a hospital is bed rails because they may be touched frequently by the patient and many healthcare providers over the course of a day, and they may not be routinely disinfected. The spores of *Clostridioides difficile* may survive for up to 5 months on inanimate surfaces, such as bed rails. Hepatitis B virus can survive up to 1 week; influenza virus can survive for 8 hours.

101. C: If venipuncture is attempted and no blood returns when the evacuated tube is attached but the needle appears to be in the vein, the initial response should be to reposition the needle. The first maneuver should be to gently pull the needle back. If this does not facilitate blood flow, then the needle may be rotated slightly in case the bevel is against the wall of the vein. Applying slight distal tension to the skin or changing the angle of needle insertion may also help. If none of these methods are effective, the evacuated tube may be defective, so it should be exchanged for another tube.

102. D: After a specimen of blood is removed from the body, the minimum time it will take to clot is generally 30 minutes for blood with appropriate clotting mechanisms. Most laboratories process serum after allowing 30 minutes (but no more than 60 minutes) for clotting. Blood clots can occur even in tubes with an anticoagulant if the tube is not inverted properly to mix the additive with the specimen. Even small clots may alter test results, so specimens should be examined prior to processing.

103. D: Sweat glands are a type of exocrine gland; exocrine glands are composed of ducts that carry secretions to the body surface or to organs. The pancreas, pituitary, and thyroid are endocrine glands, or ductless glands that secrete hormones directly into the bloodstream.

104. A: The tourniquet should be placed 5–10 cm (2–4 inches), or about 3 finger widths, superior to (above) the venipuncture site. The tourniquet should never be placed inferior to (below) the venipuncture site, as this would obstruct the flow of venous blood to the site, making blood withdrawal impossible. *Anterior* refers to something in front of something else and *posterior* means in back of something else, so these terms do not apply to tourniquet application.

105. A: The test that requires fasting for accuracy is glucose because glucose levels vary widely depending on diet and caloric intake. Other tests that usually require fasting include triglycerides and other measures of cholesterol. Panels that include glucose, such as the basic and comprehensive metabolic panels, require fasting. Fasting is recommended for a general health panel that includes CBC, CMP, and TSH. Other tests that are usually done after fasting include homocysteine, renal function tests, and tests for vitamin B12 and folate.

106. B: If a physician has ordered venipuncture for blood C&S (culture and sensitivity), CBC (complete blood count), and BMP (basic metabolic panel) for an adult patient, the correct order of draw is:

1. C&S, so that the specimen remains sterile and not contaminated by additives
2. BMP, which can be performed on plasma or serum
3. CBC, which requires whole blood for testing

107. B: If, after the phlebotomist completes a venipuncture that required fasting, the patient asks for a drink of water but none is available, the phlebotomist should refer the request to a nurse. While most fasting tests allow the patient to drink water, the patient may be on restricted intake for a number of reasons, so the phlebotomist should not administer any water to the patient if none is available at bedside for patient use.

108. C: Exercise may increase blood levels of protein, insulin, glucose, cholesterol, and skeletal muscle enzymes, but it does not affect liver enzyme levels.

109. A: *Accessioning of specimens* refers to receiving and recording specimens as they are brought to the lab. The accessioning process usually involves entering the sample into the laboratory information system and assigning and labeling it with a barcode (unless a barcode was already assigned before sample collection). An accession number is usually provided by the laboratory information system. This number helps track the sample and the testing results.

110. B: Measurement of cardiac troponin is useful in the diagnosis of acute myocardial infarction (heart attack). Glucose testing is used in diagnosing diabetes. Hematocrit is used for diagnosing anemia. Fecal occult blood is used for colon cancer screening.

111. C: Warning signs, such as "fall precautions," are usually placed on the door of an inpatient's room. The phlebotomist should always check the outside of the door for guidance. Other signs may include isolation notices or signs indicating limited visitation. If a patient has a severe allergy (such as to latex), this may also be indicated by a sign on the door. In some institutions, pictures are used instead of words for privacy reasons, so the phlebotomist should be familiar with the usual signs.

112. C: Raising the arm is not used to help visualize superficial veins. The arm may be lowered, as this helps to fill the veins. Other methods include applying warm, moist compresses to the site for 5 minutes prior to venipuncture (using care to not burn the patient), lightly massaging the vein from distal to proximal (wrist toward elbow), and lightly tapping the vein with an index or middle finger.

113. C: A FBS that is ordered QID a.c. (*ante cibum*) and h.s. (*hour of sleep*) must be done 4 times daily, before meals and at bedtime. The designation for "after meals" is p.c. (*post cibum*). "Three times daily" is abbreviated as TID (*ter in die*). While QID (*quater in die*) is often used to mean 4 times daily, it can easily be confused with QD (*quaque die*), which means "daily," so use of QID as an abbreviation is often prohibited, and written orders using this abbreviation should be questioned.

114. D: Five drops of blood are required for newborn blood spot collection on a screening card, which contains five circles for blood. The first drop of blood (usually from a heelstick) should be wiped away, then the screening card is carefully placed against the next blood drop (not pressed onto the heel) and the blood is allowed to saturate the circle. All five circles must be filled, one at a time, with only one blood drop per circle.

115. C: The type of fluid that is collected with a thoracentesis is pleural, which is fluid from the pleural cavity that surrounds the lungs. An arthrocentesis into a joint collects synovial fluid. A paracentesis (abdominocentesis) withdraws excess fluid from the peritoneal cavity of the abdomen. An amniocentesis withdraws amniotic fluid from inside the placenta. A pericardiocentesis withdraws fluid from the pericardial sac that surrounds the heart. In medical terminology, -*centesis* means to puncture and aspirate.

116. B: The act of pumping the fist during venipuncture risks a false elevation of potassium in the blood specimen, which may lead to dangerous interventions that are not only unnecessary, but can be life-threatening to the patient. For this reason, patients should never be advised to pump their fist before or during venipuncture. The patient may be advised to clench their hand in a fist to aid in site identification, and to release the fist once blood is being drawn.

117. D: The myocardial infarction (MI), or heart attack, panel does not include creatinine. The troponin test is the only test specific to cardiac muscle. Levels increase within 3–4 hours of an MI and stay elevated for 10–14 days. Myoglobin begins to increase within 2–3 hours of an MI, peaking within 8–12 hours; however, it is not specific to the heart but also found in skeletal muscle. Levels return to normal within 24 hours. Creatine kinase isoenzyme MB (CK-MB) increases within 3–4 hours, peaking at 18–24 hours and returning to normal within 72 hours.

118. C: The test that is not part of enzyme studies for a heart attack is the CK-BB (creatine kinase BB), which is found in the brain. Troponin levels are most sensitive for diagnosing a heart attack, with levels increasing within 3–12 hours of the heart attack and peaking at 24–48 hours. Myoglobin levels increase within 1–4 hours but are not specific for heart attack. CK-MB is specific to the heart and levels rise within 3–12 hours, peaking at 24 hours, but CK-MB is less sensitive and specific than troponins.

119. C: In most states, the qualifications for phlebotomists are determined by employers. Four states (California, Louisiana, Nevada, and Washington) currently require that phlebotomists meet specific qualifications, which include completing a phlebotomist training program and receiving licensure; other states are still exploring instituting requirements for education and/or licensure. Accrediting agencies generally require that phlebotomists have education and the training needed to carry out their duties. Employers may provide on-the-job training or may require that phlebotomists have certification or training before hire.

120. D: The patient's address is not required on the computer-generated requisition for a blood test. Required information includes the patient's name and birthdate (often used to verify identity), any relevant allergies/sensitivities (including latex sensitivity), test status (specific guidelines such as the need for fasting prior to testing), and the date that the test is to be done. For inpatients, the patient's room, bed, and ID numbers should also be included. For outpatients, the billing information and ICD-9 code should be included.

Practice Test #4

1. The order of the draw for specimens obtained by capillary puncture is (first to last):

- a. Other additives, EDTA, serum
- b. Serum, EDTA, other additives
- c. EDTA, serum, other additives
- d. EDTA, other additives, serum

2. After cleansing the skin for a venipuncture, the phlebotomist should NOT:

- a. Allow the antiseptic to air dry.
- b. Cleanse a second time.
- c. Wipe the skin dry.
- d. Choose an alternate site.

3. If a small bench fire occurs in the laboratory, the first step in using the portable fire extinguisher is to:

- a. Pull the pin.
- b. Hold the extinguisher in an upright position and squeeze the trigger.
- c. Remove the seal.
- d. Aim the spray nozzle at the base of the flames.

4. *Capillary action* refers to:

- a. The ability of a capillary to dilate
- b. The ability of a capillary to constrict
- c. The ability of capillaries to form a bridge between venules and arterioles
- d. The ability of a liquid to be automatically drawn into a tube without gravity or force

5. The presence of a wheal indicates:

- a. Proper injection of a local anesthetic
- b. Positive TB test
- c. Positive Allen test
- d. Improper injection of the TB antigen

6. Exchange of information contained in electronic health records is regulated by:

- a. FCC
- b. FDA
- c. HIPAA
- d. CDC

7. When collecting samples for several tests including a blood culture, the specimen for the blood culture must be collected:

- a. Whenever it is convenient
- b. Last
- c. First
- d. After the blue-capped collection tube

8. The artery that is most commonly used for arterial blood sampling is the:

   a. Radial
   b. Ulnar
   c. Brachial
   d. Axillary

9. Proper technique for needle insertion includes:

   a. Pushing down on the needle
   b. Using a C hold
   c. Using an L hold
   d. Advancing the needle slowly

10. To reduce the risk of transmission of a bloodborne pathogen via an open wound, the phlebotomist should:

   a. Cleanse the wound with bleach.
   b. Cleanse the wound with an antiseptic.
   c. Cleanse the wound with soap and water.
   d. Squeeze the wound to release fluid.

11. Lipid profiles may be completed on:

   a. Whole blood only
   b. Serum only
   c. Plasma only
   d. Serum or plasma

12. If a physician has ordered 4 different blood tests for a patient, the first thing that the phlebotomist should consider is:

   a. The time needed for venipuncture
   b. The order of draw
   c. The needle size
   d. The equipment needed

13. The most effective means of reducing the risk of infection during venipuncture is:

   a. Skin antisepsis
   b. Disinfection of environmental surfaces
   c. Handwashing
   d. Rapid processing

14. Which tube type is the most frequent source of carryover contamination?

   a. Heparin tubes
   b. EDTA tubes
   c. PTT tests
   d. Coagulation tubes

15. The document that outlines a patient's wishes about medical treatment and interventions in end-of-life care is a(n):

a. Power of attorney
b. Do-not-resuscitate directive
c. Will and testimony
d. Advance directive

16. For venipuncture with a needle and syringe, following activation of the needle safety features, the next step is to:

a. Change needles.
b. Inject the specimen into the specimen tube.
c. Attach the transfer device to the needle.
d. Remove and discard the needle.

17. If the phlebotomist notes clots in the whole blood collection tube of a sample for a PT, the phlebotomist should:

a. Transport the tube for processing.
b. Discard the tube.
c. Invert the tube 5 times.
d. Ask a supervisor for advice.

18. For blood collection with the butterfly infusion set in a child, the phlebotomist should use a:

a. 23-gauge needle with a 5-mL tube
b. 21-gauge needle with a 5-mL tube
c. 23-gauge needle with a 2-mL tube
d. 22-gauge needle with a 2-mL tube

19. Blood should never be drawn on a patient who is:

a. Unconscious
b. Confused
c. Upset
d. Asleep

20. If drawing blood from an unconscious patient, the phlebotomist should assume that the patient:

a. Will remain immobile
b. Cannot hear
c. Will move
d. Is insensate

21. Intraoperative blood collection may be used in which type of surgery?

a. Transplant
b. Cancer
c. Lower GI tract
d. Pediatric

22. A urine sample is considered acidic if its pH is:
   a. Less than 4.5
   b. Less than 7
   c. Greater than 7
   d. Greater than 8

23. If a patient complains of feeling faint and appears suddenly pale and shaky during a venipuncture, the initial response should be to:
   a. Complete the blood draw.
   b. Call for help.
   c. Remove the needle.
   d. Tell the patient to place their head between their legs.

24. All of the following statements regarding tourniquet application are true EXCEPT:
   a. The patient should be told to pump his fist.
   b. A tourniquet may be applied over the patient's sleeve.
   c. Two tourniquets may be used together.
   d. A tourniquet should not be applied over an open sore.

25. If a physician has withdrawn synovial fluid and wants to send a specimen for Gram staining, culture, and sensitivity, the collection tube should contain:
   a. Sodium heparin
   b. EDTA
   c. No additive
   d. Thrombin

26. In infants, which of the following sites may be used for arterial puncture?
   a. Brachial artery
   b. Umbilical artery
   c. Femoral artery
   d. Ulnar artery

27. The abbreviation *Q2H* in a drug order indicates that the drug should be given:
   a. Twice a day
   b. Every hour
   c. By mouth
   d. Every 2 hours

28. Which of the following is a blood test used to assess liver function?
   a. CBC
   b. Hgb
   c. AST
   d. ESR

29. When collecting a blood sample with a capillary tube, the phlebotomist should:
   a. Allow blood to flow by capillary action.
   b. Milk the puncture site.
   c. Scoop the blood into the tube.
   d. Reapply alcohol to promote blood flow.

30. Proper procedure for TB skin testing includes:

    a. Applying pressure to the site
    b. Wiping the site with gauze
    c. Avoiding areas of the arm with excessive hair
    d. Applying a bandage to the site

31. Sharps containers should never be filled more than _____ full.

    a. 50%
    b. 70%
    c. 80%
    d. 100%

32. If the phlebotomist is collecting samples for blood cultures from an adult but only 12 mL can be collected, the correct procedure is to put:

    a. 10 mL in the anaerobic tube and 2 mL in the aerobic tube
    b. 10 mL in the aerobic tube and 2 mL in the anaerobic tube
    c. 6 mL in the aerobic tube and 6 mL in the anaerobic tube
    d. 8 mL in the aerobic tube and 4 mL in the anaerobic tube

33. If a phlebotomist is exposed to blood containing HIV, PEP must be started within _____ to be effective.

    a. 72 hours
    b. 1 week
    c. 2 weeks
    d. 3 weeks

34. Which of the following tests is an example of an immunologic test?

    a. LD
    b. RF
    c. BUN
    d. MCH

35. When the phlebotomist is taking collection tubes with blood specimens from an isolation room, the specimens should be:

    a. Sealed in a leak-proof plastic bag
    b. Covered with a sterile drape
    c. Placed in a labeled paper bag
    d. Transported as usual

36. The hemoglobin A1c POC test reflects the average blood glucose level for the previous:

    a. 2–3 days
    b. 7–10 days
    c. 4–5 weeks
    d. 2–3 months

37. An indication that a localized infection has progressed to septicemia is:
  a. Chills and fever
  b. Erythema
  c. Localized edema
  d. Bradycardia

38. Therapeutic phlebotomy is used for all of the following EXCEPT:
  a. Polycythemia
  b. Toxicology studies
  c. Hemochromatosis
  d. Sickle cell anemia

39. Which of the following laboratory tests often shows decreased values in older adults?
  a. Hct
  b. RBC count
  c. WBC count
  d. Creatinine clearance

40. If a patient is extremely obese and the phlebotomist cannot palpate or locate the veins in the arms, the best solution is to:
  a. Call for assistance.
  b. Estimate vein position and attempt venipuncture.
  c. Request a change to an arterial blood draw.
  d. Use foot or ankle veins.

41. To prevent transmission of pathogenic organisms, natural nails should NOT be longer than:
  a. 1/16 inch
  b. 1/8 inch
  c. 1/4 inch
  d. 1/2 inch

42. If the phlebotomist has made two unsuccessful attempts to draw blood from a patient, the next step should be to:
  a. Utilize an assistive device for the next attempt.
  b. Wait 5 minutes before the next attempt.
  c. Call for another phlebotomist or notify the physician.
  d. Notify the supervisor.

43. If, when the phlebotomist arrives in a patient's room to do a blood draw, the patient says that the physician advised her that she would need no further blood tests, the phlebotomist should:
  a. Assure the patient that the physician ordered the tests.
  b. Ask when the physician made the statement.
  c. Assume that the patient is incorrect.
  d. Verify the orders with the physician.

44. Which type of lancet is most likely indicated when the phlebotomist needs to fill multiple microcollection tubes?

    a. Blade, 2 mm × 1.5 mm
    b. Blade, 1 mm × 1.5 mm
    c. Needle, 28-gauge
    d. Needle, 23 gauge

45. Which of the following tests is NOT included in the BMP?

    a. Glucose
    b. Potassium
    c. BUN
    d. Triglycerides

46. In a laboratory, the job of the cytotechnologist is to:

    a. Prepare samples of body tissues for examination.
    b. Examine body cells to detect and stage cancer.
    c. Perform general laboratory tests.
    d. Examine tissues and interpret laboratory results.

47. What is the purpose of the gel in the plasma separator tube?

    a. Providing anticoagulation
    b. Separating plasma from cells
    c. Preventing contamination
    d. Speeding clotting

48. Under which of the following conditions is underfilling additive tubes NOT acceptable?

    a. When drawing blood from children
    b. When drawing blood from anemic patients
    c. When using a red top or SST
    d. As a time-saving strategy

49. Which of the following statements regarding HBV is FALSE?

    a. The HBV vaccine also protects against HDV.
    b. The HBV vaccine does not contain live virus.
    c. The HBV vaccine may pose a risk of HBV transmission.
    d. HBV can survive up to 1 week in dried blood.

50. In which of the following patients is blood collection prohibited?

    a. Patient with a hematoma in the antecubital area of each arm
    b. Pregnant patient
    c. Mastectomy patient
    d. Patient with full sleeve tattoos

51. A patient's blood glucose level is usually elevated:

    a. After fasting
    b. After ingesting a low-carbohydrate meal
    c. After ingesting a high-carbohydrate meal
    d. Two hours after ingesting a high-carbohydrate meal

52. To aliquot a specimen means to:

    a. Divide the specimen into portions.
    b. Dilute the specimen.
    c. Concentrate the specimen.
    d. Centrifuge the specimen.

53. The closure cap of the collection tube that has been specifically designed to meet AABB requirements is:

    a. Lavender
    b. Yellow
    c. Pink
    d. Navy blue

54. *Pre-* and *post-* are examples of:

    a. Abbreviations
    b. Suffixes
    c. Prefixes
    d. Root words

55. When selecting a vein for venipuncture, you should:

    a. Select a vein close to a pulse.
    b. Use the basilic vein as an alternative if the median cubital vein cannot be located.
    c. Palpate visible veins.
    d. Use your thumb to palpate a vein.

56. Handwritten patient ID labels are often used instead of preprinted labels for:

    a. Blood bank testing
    b. Cost savings
    c. Genetic testing
    d. C&S

57. If the cord of a piece of equipment is frayed, the appropriate initial action is to:

    a. Apply tape to the frayed area.
    b. Unplug the equipment.
    c. Call for service.
    d. Notify a supervisor.

58. When using a bariatric blood pressure cuff instead of a tourniquet for an obese patient, the blood pressure cuff should be inflated to:

    a. Just above the patient's systolic pressure
    b. Just below the patient's systolic pressure
    c. Just above the patient's diastolic pressure
    d. Just below the patient's diastolic pressure

59. The active safety device on a double-pointed needle is generally activated by:

    a. Pulling backward with the thumb
    b. Pulling backward with the index finger
    c. Pushing forward with the thumb
    d. Pushing forward with the index finger

60. Newborn screening should be carried out after the first _____ of life.

   a. 12 hours
   b. 18 hours
   c. 24 hours
   d. 48 hours

61. If a vein collapses during a blood draw, the initial action should be to:

   a. Rotate the needle.
   b. Insert the needle further into the vein.
   c. Apply pressure above the venipuncture site.
   d. Slightly withdraw the needle.

62. Which of the following statements regarding the aPTT test is FALSE?

   a. Plasma values of approximately 30–40 seconds are considered normal.
   b. Samples must be frozen.
   c. It is used to monitor the effectiveness of heparin therapy.
   d. Samples must be processed more quickly for patients on heparin therapy than for other patients.

63. If drawing blood from a metacarpal vein, the tourniquet should be placed 3–4 inches:

   a. Above the elbow
   b. Below the elbow
   c. Above the wrist bone
   d. Below the wrist bone

64. A condition characterized by protrusion of the stomach through a weak area of the diaphragm is known as:

   a. Gastritis
   b. GERD
   c. Hiatal hernia
   d. Peptic ulcer

65. If a patient is chewing gum while the phlebotomist prepares to draw blood for a CBC, the patient should be:

   a. Allowed to continue
   b. Asked to remove the gum
   c. Asked to refrain from actively chewing during the procedure
   d. Asked if the gum is sugar free

66. If, after leaving a patient's room, the phlebotomist is asked by the patient's brother what tests the patient is having, the phlebotomist should:

   a. Provide information.
   b. Provide no information.
   c. Deny having any knowledge.
   d. Ask the patient's permission to divulge information.

67. All of the following may trigger hematoma formation EXCEPT:

    a. Venipuncture into small veins
    b. Inadequate pressure to the venipuncture site after the needle is removed
    c. Needle penetration all the way through the vein
    d. Petechiae

68. PEP after needlestick injury is available for:

    a. HIV and HCV
    b. HIV and HBV
    c. HBV and HCV
    d. HIV only

69. Labeling a tube after collection of a blood sample should be done:

    a. In the patient's presence
    b. After leaving the patient's presence
    c. After entering the laboratory
    d. Before placing the tubes for processing

70. Following venipuncture with excessive bleeding, a saturated bloodstained gauze should be placed in a:

    a. Paper bag
    b. Hazardous waste container
    c. Bedside wastebasket
    d. Sharps container

71. Which of the following tests is most often used to monitor unfractionated heparin therapy?

    a. APTT
    b. INR
    c. PT
    d. TT

72. If an antecubital vein cannot be located, you may:

    a. Use a vein on the underside of the wrist.
    b. Perform a capillary puncture.
    c. Manipulate the site until a vein can be found.
    d. Use a tendon.

73. Which of the following statements regarding healthcare communication is FALSE?

    a. Comfort zones are dependent on culture.
    b. Callers should not be put on hold.
    c. Sign language may be used for hearing-impaired patients.
    d. Medical interpreters may be used for non–English-speaking patients.

74. How frequently must medical facilities review the availability of safer medical devices?

    a. Monthly
    b. Every 6 months
    c. Annually
    d. Every 2 years

75. If blood must be drawn from a 3-year-old child, the phlebotomist should:

   a. Ask the parent to wait outside the room.
   b. Explain the procedure to the parent only.
   c. Ask a nurse to hold the child.
   d. Explain the procedure to the child.

76. If, when the phlebotomist is performing a venipuncture in the antecubital space, the patient grabs the arm and complains of severe, shock-like shooting pain, the initial response should be to:

   a. Complete the blood collection.
   b. Remove the needle and apply pressure.
   c. Reassure the patient.
   d. Remove the needle and apply ice.

77. A standard blood specimen should be transported:

   a. In a biohazard bag at room temperature
   b. In a clear bag on ice
   c. In a biohazard bag on ice
   d. In a sterile container that is puncture-proof

78. An outpatient's blood should NOT be drawn:

   a. While the patient is reclining in a chair
   b. While the patient is lying down
   c. Unless the patient is seated in a blood-drawing chair
   d. While the patient is seated on a stool

79. At room temperature, EDTA specimens for ESR should be tested within:

   a. 1 hour
   b. 2 hours
   c. 4 hours
   d. 6 hours

80. In a hospital environment, infection is most commonly spread by:

   a. Contaminated equipment
   b. The ventilation system
   c. Contaminated hands
   d. Contaminated food

81. Which of the following is NOT a cause of vein collapse?

   a. Tourniquet too close to the venipuncture site
   b. Vacuum draw of the tube
   c. Stoppage of blood flow on tourniquet removal
   d. Frequent venipunctures

82. Hydrocephalus is characterized by:

   a. Stiff neck
   b. Nerve pain
   c. Shuffling gait
   d. Enlarged head

83. **For which of the following tests must the blood specimen be immediately chilled?**

   a. Hematocrit
   b. Cryofibrinogen
   c. Cold agglutinins
   d. Lactic acid

84. **Specimens for which of the following tests require centrifugation?**

   a. Hemoglobin A1c
   b. CBC
   c. Cyclosporine
   d. Cholesterol

85. **Which of the following is a characteristic of negligence?**

   a. Intent to harm
   b. Invasion of privacy
   c. Injury
   d. Abandonment

86. **Protective isolation may be required for all of the following patients EXCEPT:**

   a. Neutropenic chemotherapy patients
   b. Burn patients
   c. Infants
   d. AIDS patients

87. **Standard precautions must be used with:**

   a. All patients
   b. Patients with infections
   c. Immunocompromised patients
   d. Hospitalized patients

88. **Which of the following tests are NOT usually part of the workup for DIC, a coagulation disorder?**

   a. Hgb and Hct
   b. PT, aPTT, and TT
   c. D-dimer and fibrinogen
   d. ESR and BUN

89. **If using a BP cuff instead of a tourniquet for venipuncture, the BP cuff should NOT be inflated to more than:**

   a. 20 mmHg
   b. 40 mmHg
   c. Slightly below the individual's baseline diastolic blood pressure
   d. Slightly below the individual's baseline systolic blood pressure

90. When drawing blood from a patient with moderate to advanced dementia, it is most important to:

a. Use minimal supplies.
b. Explain the procedure.
c. Work quickly.
d. Ask for assistance.

91. Which of the following tests requires that the specimen be protected from light?

a. Testosterone
b. Vitamin D
c. Creatinine
d. Bilirubin

92. Which of the following positions is usually the best for a toddler who needs a venipuncture?

a. Supine
b. Side-lying
c. Prone with arm extended
d. Hug hold, facing the parent

93. The source of transmission of a pathogen to others is known as the:

a. Susceptible host
b. Reservoir host
c. Direct contact
d. Chain of infection

94. Which of the following vaccinations is NOT routinely recommended for phlebotomists?

a. HBV
b. MMR
c. Influenza
d. HZV

95. Which of the following statements regarding patient identification is FALSE?

a. An outpatient may be identified by an ID card.
b. An outpatient should be asked to state his or her name and date of birth.
c. If a patient has been identified by the receptionist, no further verification is needed.
d. A patient's response when his or her name is called is not sufficient for identification.

96. Bandages are usually avoided in children younger than 2 years because:

a. They are not needed.
b. Toddlers often have latex allergies.
c. They may cause contact dermatitis.
d. They pose a choking hazard.

97. Which of the following information is NOT required on specimen tube labels?

a. Accession number
b. Physician's signature
c. Phlebotomist's initials
d. Time of test

98. If the laboratory protocol calls for the use of chlorhexidine solution for skin antisepsis for skin puncture or venipuncture, the antiseptic should NOT be used on infants younger than:

    a. 12 months
    b. 6 months
    c. 4 months
    d. 2 months

99. The ACT test is used to monitor:

    a. pO_2
    b. Heparin
    c. Ionized calcium
    d. Glucose

100. When performing venipuncture on a patient with extensive burns, the phlebotomist should:

    a. Pad the tourniquet area.
    b. Avoid burned areas.
    c. Use a winged infusion set.
    d. Avoid using a tourniquet.

101. A decreased blood level of which of the following causes an increase in respiration rate?

    a. pCO_2
    b. pO_2
    c. HCO_3
    d. pH

102. If plasma is needed for a chemistry test, the blood may be collected in a tube containing:

    a. Sodium heparin
    b. Potassium chloride
    c. EDTA
    d. Clot activator

103. Which of the following tests may be performed together to assess clotting abnormalities?

    a. ACT and PT
    b. ACT and aPTT
    c. PT and PTT
    d. PT and PP

104. Which of the following is required for drug or alcohol testing?

    a. Patient consent
    b. Split sample
    c. Glass tube
    d. Blood and urine samples

105. PPE is NOT required when entering the room of a patient with:
   a. Skin infection
   b. Tuberculosis
   c. Intestinal infection
   d. HIV

106. If a patient states he has severe needle phobia, the phlebotomist should:
   a. Have the patient lie flat for venipuncture.
   b. Reassure the patient that the venipuncture will not hurt.
   c. Tell the patient to take deep breaths.
   d. Reassure the patient that the procedure is very fast.

107. A phlebotomist who wears contact lenses should:
   a. Avoid wearing them in the laboratory.
   b. Wear only hard lenses.
   c. Wear only soft lenses.
   d. Wear protective goggles in the laboratory.

108. All of the following are skin tests EXCEPT:
   a. PPD
   b. Histoplasma
   c. BNP
   d. Coccidioidal

109. Which of the following methods may prevent hemoconcentration during a venipuncture?
   a. Ask the patient to hold a fist during blood flow.
   b. Thoroughly massage the vein prior to venipuncture.
   c. Release the tourniquet with 2 minutes.
   d. Advise the patient to avoid pumping their fist.

110. An increased eosinophil count often indicates a(n):
   a. Viral infection
   b. Vascular trauma
   c. Allergic reaction
   d. Bacterial infection

111. A safe area for capillary puncture in infants is the:
   a. Medial plantar surface of the heel
   b. Posterior curvature of the heel
   c. Arch of the foot
   d. Earlobe

112. Which of the following specimens must be kept at or near body temperature?
   a. Lactic acid
   b. Ammonia
   c. Glucagon
   d. Cryoglobulin

113. A patient hospitalized for chemotherapy for renal cancer would most likely be treated in which department?

    a. Oncology
    b. Hematology
    c. Endocrinology
    d. Cardiology

114. Blood levels of which of the following are normally lowest in the morning?

    a. Iron
    b. Insulin
    c. Potassium
    d. Glucose

115. To prevent hemoconcentration during venipuncture, the phlebotomist should:

    a. Massage the area until a vein is located.
    b. Ask the patient to release his or her fist when blood flow begins.
    c. Ask the patient to vigorously pump his or her fist.
    d. Redirect the needle several times until a vein is located.

116. Which type of microorganism is usually the causative agent in sepsis?

    a. Viruses
    b. Parasites
    c. Fungi
    d. Bacteria

117. When collecting a blood specimen from a 2-month-old infant, the primary interactions will be between the phlebotomist and the:

    a. Infant
    b. Nurse
    c. Parent
    d. Physician

118. According to the order of draw, which collection tube/bottle should be filled first?

    a. Light-blue–capped tube
    b. Green-capped tube
    c. Red-and-black–capped tube
    d. Blood culture bottle

119. The white blood cell type that is most likely to increase in number in response to bacterial infection is the:

    a. Monocyte
    b. Basophil
    c. Eosinophil
    d. Neutrophil

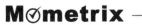

120. All of the following are used to send laboratory requisition forms to the lab EXCEPT:

    a.   Courier
    b.   Pneumatic tubes
    c.   E-mail
    d.   Verbal laboratory request

Answer Key and Explanations for Test #4

1. D: The order of the draw for specimens obtained by capillary puncture is (first to last) EDTA specimens, specimens requiring other additives, then serum specimens. Puncturing the skin begins the coagulation process because the body responds to trauma with hemostasis and clotting, so the specimens should be obtained quickly, with the EDTA specimen collected first because this specimen will be used for hematology studies and will be the most affected by clotting.

2. C: After cleansing the skin for a venipuncture, the phlebotomist should not wipe the skin dry, but rather should allow the skin to air dry completely, which will take about 30 seconds. There is no prohibition against cleansing the skin a second time, and this may be necessary if the site is inadvertently contaminated. Applying the wet antiseptic is sometimes helpful in visualizing the vein, and the phlebotomist may choose an alternate site at any time.

3. A: If a small bench fire occurs in the laboratory, the first step in using the portable fire extinguisher is to pull the pin. The acronym PASS stands for the following:

- **P**ull the pin.
- **A**im the spray nozzle at the base of the flames.
- **S**queeze the trigger while holding the extinguisher in an upright position.
- **S**weep the spray nozzle from side to side to cover the area of the fire with the spray.

4. D: *Capillary action* refers to the ability of a liquid to be automatically drawn into a tube without gravity or force. Capillary tubes and microhematocrit tubes fill by capillary action, and blood will rise into the tubes if they are held vertically to the blood drop, or blood will flow into the tubes if they are held horizontally to the blood drop. The end of the tube must stay at the drop and should not be moved because air may enter the tube, which may interfere with the test results.

5. A: The presence of a wheal, or bleb, indicates proper injection of a local anesthetic prior to arterial puncture. A wheal also serves as indication of proper injection of the antigen during tuberculosis (TB) testing. A induration, or area of hardened tissue, indicates a positive TB reaction. A positive Allen test is indicated by the hand flushing pink or regaining normal coloration within 15 seconds.

6. C: Exchange of information contained in electronic health records (EHRs) is regulated by HIPAA (Health Insurance Portability and Accountability Act). HIPAA mandates both privacy and security rules to ensure that all information contained in the EHR remains confidential with methods in place to limit access. Electronic health information must be safeguarded through security methods to ensure that non-permitted disclosures do not occur. Only those authorized to access a patient's EHR may do so.

7. C: When collecting samples for several tests including a blood culture, the specimen for the blood culture must be collected first to avoid possible contamination of the specimen. Blood culture collection tubes may vary in shape and color of cap, but all culture collection tubes contain media that promotes growth of microorganisms. Skin must be carefully cleansed with antiseptics prior to venipuncture so that bacteria on the surface of the skin do not contaminate the sample.

8. A: The artery that is most commonly used for arterial blood sampling is the radial artery, which branches off of the brachial artery on the thumb side. The radial artery lies relatively close to the surface, so it is easier to access than arteries that are deeper in tissue. The ulnar artery also branches off of the brachial artery, but on the opposite (little finger) side. Arteries are oxygen-carrying vessels and are used primarily for blood gases because the levels of gases and the pH of the arterial blood are critically important.

9. C: The proper technique for anchoring the vein before venipuncture is known as the L hold technique. It involves using the fingers to support the back of the patient's arm below the elbow and placing the thumb 1 to 2 inches below and slightly to the side of the venipuncture site to pull the patient's skin toward the wrist. The C hold technique, or the two-finger technique, should not be used because it may result in the needle springing back into the phlebotomist's index finger if the patient pulls his or her arm back. Pushing down on the needle during insertion is painful and may increase the risk of blood leakage. Advancing the needle too slowly may prolong the patient's discomfort.

10. C: Cleansing the wound with plain soap and water for at least 30 seconds is useful in reducing the risk of transmission of a bloodborne pathogen via an open wound. Squeezing the wound or cleansing the wound with an antiseptic, bleach, or other caustic agent is not recommended.

11. D: Lipid (fat) profiles may be completed with serum or plasma. A lipid profile (also called a cholesterol study) is done to evaluate a patient's risk of coronary artery disease, heart attack (myocardial infarction), and stroke (cerebrovascular accident [CVA]). Patients are advised to fast for 12 hours prior to the test except for water, coffee, or tea (no milk, cream, or sugar). The lipid profile includes HDL (high-density lipoprotein), LDL (low-density lipoprotein), triglycerides, total cholesterol, and total cholesterol/HDL ratio (optimal is 3.5:1).

12. B: If a physician has ordered 4 different blood tests for a patient, the first thing that the phlebotomist should consider is the order of draw because this helps to determine which evacuated tubes and other equipment is needed and ensures that the proper order is followed. The needle size should be determined after the patient is examined and the phlebotomist is able to assess the person's veins. The blood collection tray should contain needles in different sizes as well as winged ("butterfly") infusion sets.

13. C: While skin antisepsis and disinfection of environmental surfaces are important, the most effective means of reducing the risk of infection during venipuncture is actually handwashing because contact with dirty hands is the mode by which infections are most easily passed from one person to another. The phlebotomist should wash their hands with soap and water or alcohol-based hand rub before beginning the venipuncture (and before applying gloves) and should again wash their hands when the procedure is completed.

14. B: EDTA tubes are more frequently associated with carryover contamination than any other types of additives, while heparin is associated with the least amount of interference. Coagulation tubes, which contain sodium citrate, are the first to be filled because all other additives interfere with coagulation tests. Partial thromboplastin time (PTT) tests are affected by tissue thromboplastin contamination.

15. D: The document that outlines a patient's wishes about medical treatment and interventions in end-of-life care is an advance directive. Laws regarding advance directives vary somewhat from one state to another, but in most states they are not binding and may be overruled by family members if the patient is unable to indicate preferences. People should always inform family members and healthcare providers about their wishes and provide copies of the advance directive, which may contain a do-not-resuscitate order.

16. D: Immediately following venipuncture with a needle and syringe, the first step is to activate needle safety features while the needle is still in the arm or immediately after it is removed, depending on the manufacturer's instructions. Then, remove and discard the needle. Next, the hub of the needle is attached to the transfer device. With the syringe tip-down in a vertical position and the transfer device at the bottom, the collection tube is inserted into the transfer device. The tube must fill by vacuum draw and not through depressing the plunger because using the plunger can cause hemolysis of the sample. Once all of the necessary tubes are filled, the syringe and the transfer device are disposed of together (do not separate) into a sharps container.

17. B: Since the PT (prothrombin time) evaluates clotting time, if clots are present in the sample prior to processing, the sample should be discarded and another blood sample drawn because the results will not be accurate. Whole blood specimens for PT must be maintained at room temperature and may be stored for up to 24 hours, although if other coagulation tests, such as the aPTT (non-heparinized) will be run on the sample, it can only be stored for up to 4 hours; heparinized samples can be stored for a maximum of 1 hour.

18. C: For a pediatric patient, a 23-gauge needle with a 2-mL tube should be used for blood collection using a butterfly infusion set. Use of a 5-mL tube with a 23-gauge needle may cause vein collapse or hemolysis of the specimen.

19. D: Blood should never be drawn on a patient who is asleep because the patient may react violently or move abruptly, putting both the phlebotomist and the patient at risk for injury. In addition, the phlebotomist must wake the patient and explain the procedure, as there is no implied consent otherwise. Many patients may be confused, upset, or even unconscious, and while blood can be drawn from these patients, the phlebotomist may need to take precautions, including asking for assistance, in these cases.

20. C: If drawing blood from an unconscious patient, the phlebotomist should assume that the patient will move, and so should be proactive in asking for assistance from nursing staff to immobilize the puncture site, such as by holding the arm. Many patients who appear to be unconscious still retain the ability to hear, so the phlebotomist should explain the procedure before beginning and continue describing actions during the blood draw. Unconscious patients may also experience pain and discomfort.

21. A: Intraoperative blood collection is used for procedures in which the estimated amount of blood loss is 20% or more of the patient's blood volume. The blood is collected from the incision site, filtered, washed, and returned to the patient via an IV; it is a form of autotransfusion. It is typically used in patients undergoing cardiac, vascular, gynecologic, trauma, or transplant surgery. Intraoperative blood collection is not used for cancer or lower GI tract surgery or for infants or small children due to the risk of anemia or cardiac arrest.

22. B: All aqueous (water-based) solutions have a pH, which is the negative logarithm of the concentration of hydrogen ions. The solution is considered acidic at a pH of less than 7 and alkaline (or basic) at a pH of greater than 7. Because urine is a water-based solution, the same definitions apply. Urine is therefore considered acidic if its pH is less than 7. Urine is typically acidic, but can also be alkaline; the normal pH range for urine is 4.5–8.

23. C: If a patient complains of feeling faint and appears suddenly pale and shaky during a venipuncture, the initial response should be to remove the needle because, if the patient faints and falls, it could dislodge the needle and result in trauma. As soon as the needle is removed, sitting patients should be assisted to put their heads low, between their legs. If the patient is in bed, the head of the bed should be lowered. The patient may need time to recuperate before another venipuncture is attempted.

24. A: When applying a tourniquet, fist pumping should be discouraged, as it may make vein location more difficult or cause changes in blood components that may affect test results. A tourniquet may be applied over a patient's sleeve if the sleeve is too tight and cannot be rolled up far enough. Because a tourniquet may have a tendency to roll or twist on the arm of an obese patient, two tourniquets may be stacked and used together. A tourniquet should never be placed over an open sore.

25. A: If a physician has withdrawn synovial fluid and wants to send a specimen for Gram staining, culture, and sensitivity, the collection tube should contain sodium heparin. This holds true for most bodily fluids (as opposed to blood). For cell counts, differential, and cytology, tubes should contain EDTA or sodium heparin. If testing is for glucose, protein, amylase, dehydrogenase, or other chemical tests, the tube should have no additive. Specimens should be transported to the laboratory as quickly as possible for processing.

26. B: In infants, the scalp or umbilical artery may be used for arterial puncture. The brachial artery is not used in infants or children because it is more difficult to palpate and lacks collateral circulation. The femoral artery is generally only used in emergency situations or if no other sites are available. The ulnar artery is not used for arterial puncture.

27. D: In this context, the letter *Q* stands for "every" and H stands for "hour." Therefore, *Q2H* means that the drug should be given every 2 hours. *BID* indicates that the drug should be administered twice a day, and *PO* (from the Latin *per os*) means given orally, or by mouth.

28. C: A test for the level of the enzyme aspartate aminotransferase (AST) is typically used to assess liver function, usually as part of a liver panel; a liver panel also includes ALT, ASP, bilirubin, and more. Hemoglobin (Hgb), complete blood count (CBC), and erythrocyte sedimentation rate (ESR) are used to diagnose blood diseases such as anemia or leukemia.

29. A: When collecting a blood sample with a capillary tube, the phlebotomist should allow blood to flow by capillary action, being careful to touch the end of the tube to the blood drop only. Any interference with the blood flow, such as by scooping or milking the puncture site, may cause hemolysis. After the blood is collected, pressure must be applied to the site for 2–3 minutes with the extremity elevated above the level of the heart.

30. C: When administering a tuberculosis (TB) skin test, avoid areas of the arm with scars, bruises, burns, or excessive hair because they may interfere with test results. Applying pressure to the site may force the antigen out of the site, while wiping the site with gauze may cause the antigen to be absorbed. Applying a bandage to the site may result in fluid absorption or irritation and may affect test results.

31. C: Sharps containers should never be filled more than 80% full to ensure that no material protrudes from the container or damages the container. Overfilling may make it difficult to secure the lid for disposal and may increase risk of needlesticks for those handling the container. Most containers have a line to indicate when the container is full and must be replaced. Care should be taken to avoid placing biohazardous materials, such as bloodstained gauze, into the sharps container, as these materials may prevent needles from falling to the bottom of the container.

32. B: If the phlebotomist is collecting samples for blood cultures from an adult but only 12 mL can be collected, the correct procedure is to fill the aerobic collection tube to the minimum volume recommended per tube for adults (10 mL), and then put the remaining blood in the anaerobic tube. In this case, the remaining 2 mL would be collected in the anaerobic tube.

33. A: If a phlebotomist is exposed to blood containing HIV, PEP (post-exposure prophylaxis) must be started within 72 hours in order to be effective, according to protocols established by the CDC. While treatment protocols may vary depending on the patient's viral load and other risk factors, a 4-week regimen of two or three antiretroviral drugs, such as zidovudine and lamivudine, is common. If the patient source has a drug-resistant infection, prophylaxis must be based on the drugs to which the virus is responsive.

34. B: The RF (rheumatoid factor) test is an immunologic test done to help diagnose rheumatoid arthritis, which is an autoimmune disorder. RF is an autoantibody that combines with immunoglobulin (another antibody) to cause disease. MCHC (mean corpuscular hemoglobin concentration) is a hematological test, part of the CBC (complete blood count). BUN (blood urea nitrogen) is a kidney function test. The LD (lactate dehydrogenase) test is a chemistry test of LD, which is a substance that increases with heart attack as well as chronic liver, lung, and kidney disease.

35. A: When the phlebotomist is taking collection tubes with blood specimens from an isolation room, the specimens should be sealed in a leak-proof plastic bag. A notice should be posted on each isolation room outlining the type of isolation and the requirements for PPE. The phlebotomist must always follow these guidelines and must enter wearing gloves, and should not take the phlebotomy tray into the room. Additionally, after the venipuncture and specimen collection is completed, all equipment except for the specimen containers must be left in the room in appropriate containers.

36. D: The hemoglobin A1c point-of-care (POC) test reflects the average blood glucose level for the previous 2–3 months. Glucose attaches to hemoglobin A in RBCs and remains for the life of the cells. The typical life of an RBC is approximately 120 days. Hemoglobin A1c is a better predictor of glucose control and the possibility of diabetes complications than serum glucose is. The normal value for hemoglobin A1c is less than 5.7%.

37. A: An indication that a localized infection, which is characterized by erythema (redness), edema (swelling), and localized pain, has progressed to septicemia is a sudden onset of chills and fever. Patients may exhibit tachycardia (rapid heart rate) and tachypnea (rapid breathing) as well as nausea and vomiting. Without treatment, the patient may progress to confusion and coagulation disorders characterized by ecchymosis (bruising) and petechiae (red spots) on skin. Typical diagnostic studies include blood C&S, blood gases, CBC, and clotting studies.

38. B: Therapeutic phlebotomy is the withdrawal of large volumes of blood as a treatment for certain conditions, including polycythemia, hemochromatosis, and sickle cell disease. It is not used for toxicology, which is the study of toxins or poisons.

39. D: The laboratory test that often shows decreased values in older adults is creatinine clearance, which usually decreases by about 10 mL/min each decade. There is no appreciable normal difference in RBC count, WBC count, Hgb, or Hct. Other tests that may show decreased values in older adults include total calcium, HDL, magnesium, free testosterone, aldosterone, interleukin-1, phosphorus, creatine kinase, and estradiol. Laboratory tests that often show increased age-associated values include ANA, 2-hour postprandial glucose, interleukin, PTH, PSA, ESR, triglycerides, uric acid, and rheumatoid factor.

40. A: Any time a phlebotomist is unable to palpate or locate a vein for venipuncture, they should call for assistance from someone with more experience and should not blindly attempt to do a venipuncture because this may cause unnecessary trauma. The phlebotomist may try applying a warm, moist compresses for 5 minutes to distend the veins or try using a blood pressure cuff instead of a tourniquet. A longer needle may be required, and the needle insertion angle may need to be steeper than usual because of the depth of the veins.

41. C: Per CDC guidelines, in order to prevent transmission of pathogenic organisms, natural nails should not be longer than 1/4 inch because bacteria can collect under the tip of the nail. Artificial nails should not be worn by healthcare providers with direct patient contact because of the risk of spreading infectious organisms, especially gram-negative organisms. While freshly applied nail polish does not increase risk, chipped nail polish may harbor pathogenic organisms. Handwashing alone is not sufficient to remove the bacteria associated with long and/or artificial nails.

42. C: If the phlebotomist has made two unsuccessful attempts to draw blood from a patient, CLSI guidelines recommend that the next step should be to call for another phlebotomist or to notify the physician. Making further attempts is likely to cause increased stress on the part of both the patient and the phlebotomist. Nurses can also be consulted for the next attempt. Applying warm compresses may help to make veins more visible, and assistive devices such as vein finders may be required.

43. D: If, when the phlebotomist arrives in a patient's room to do a blood draw, the patient says that the physician advised her that she would need no further blood tests, the phlebotomist should verify the orders with the physician. There is a question of informed consent because the patient does not understand why the test should be conducted. Continuing to do the blood draw without first verifying the order with the physician and providing updated information about the physician's orders may violate a patient's right to refuse treatment.

44. A: The lancet most likely indicated when the phlebotomist needs to fill multiple microcollection tubes is the 2 mm × 1.5 mm blade because it results in a higher blood flow in comparison to the others. Both the 28-gauge and the 23-gauge needles usually provide only a single drop of blood. Blades result in blood flow, but the 1 mm × 1.5 mm blade has a low flow, usually enough to provide a drop of blood or to fill a microhematocrit tube. The 1.5 mm × 1.5 mm blade provides a medium blood flow and should fill a single microcollection tube.

45. D: The test that is not included in the BMP (basic metabolic panel) is triglycerides. The BMP consists of 8 different tests that provide information about the patient's blood glucose, electrolytes, and kidney function. Tests include glucose and the electrolytes Ca (calcium), Na (sodium), K (potassium), and CO_2/HCO_3 (carbon dioxide, bicarbonate). Kidney function tests include BUN (blood urea nitrogen), which measures waste products that result from protein metabolism, and serum creatinine, which measures waste products produced by skeletal muscles.

46. B: A cytotechnologist examines body cells to detect and stage cancer. A histotechnologist prepares samples of body tissues for examination under a microscope, sometimes while the patient is undergoing surgery to help guide excision. A pathologist examines tissues and interprets laboratory results, which assists in diagnosis. This person is a physician who has specialized in pathology. Pathologists may also do postmortem examinations. A laboratory technician performs general laboratory tests.

47. B: The purpose of the gel in the plasma separator tube (light-green top) is to provide a barrier that separates the plasma from the cells during and after centrifugation. After the specimen is collected in the tube, the tube should be inverted at least 8 times. The gel rises during the centrifugation process, which usually takes about 10 minutes, as the cells separate. The barrier remains stable for 48 hours, the recommended maximum storage time.

48. D: Underfilling additive tubes as a time-saving device is unacceptable. Underfilling is acceptable when obtaining larger amounts of blood is inadvisable, such as when drawing blood from infants, children, or severely anemic adults. Short-draw serum tubes such as red tops and serum separator tubes (SSTs) are acceptable provided that the specimen is not hemolyzed and there is enough of the specimen for testing.

49. C: The HBV vaccine does not contain live virus and thus does not carry the risk of HBV infection. HBV vaccine also protects against hepatitis D virus (HDV) because HDV is only contracted concurrently with HBV. HBV can survive up to 1 week in dried blood on work surfaces or other objects.

50. A: Venipuncture should never be performed through a hematoma. If blood must be drawn from an arm with a hematoma, an area distal to the hematoma should be used. In patients with full sleeve tattoos, it is best to choose a site that does not contain any tattoo ink, but blood can be collected from a tattooed site as long as the tattoo has fully healed. In a mastectomy patient, blood should not be drawn from the arm on the same side of the mastectomy, but can be drawn from the other arm. Pregnancy does not preclude blood collection.

51. C: A patient's blood glucose level is normally elevated after ingestion of a high-carbohydrate meal; however, glucose levels return to normal within 2 hours after ingestion.

52. A: To aliquot a specimen means to divide the specimen into smaller portions. For example, if a 24-hour urine specimen has been sent to the lab for processing, any additive needed is added to the entire specimen (according to the volume) but only a small portion of that whole may be then used for testing. Part or all of the remaining volume is kept until the aliquoted specimen has been processed in case a backup specimen is required.

53. C: The closure top of the collection tube that has been specifically designed to meet AABB (American Association of Blood Banks) requirements for blood banks is pink. The pink-capped tube is essentially the same as the lavender-capped tube, as both contain EDTA as an anticoagulant, but the label for the pink-capped tube meets AABB specifications regarding patient identification. Once the specimen is collected, it is important to mix it well (inverting at least 8 times) to prevent clotting.

54. C: *Pre-* and *post-* are examples of prefixes, which are added to the beginning of a word to indicate an amount, location, or time. *Pre-* means "before" and *post-* means "after." A suffix is added to the end of a word. In medicine, the suffix may indicate a procedure, condition, or disease, such as *-algia*, which means "pain." An abbreviation is used to shorten a term. One example common in medicine is *BID*, which is an abbreviation of the Latin phrase *bis in die* and means "twice a day." A root word is the basis of a term and establishes its meaning; for example, *cardi* is a root word meaning "heart."

55. C: In selecting a vein for venipuncture, even visible veins should be palpated to judge suitability for venipuncture. If the median cubital vein cannot be located, the basilic vein should not be used unless no other vein is more prominent because of the possibility of nerve injury or damage to the brachial artery. Do not use veins that overlie or are located close to a pulse to avoid the risk of puncturing an artery. The thumb should not be used because it has a pulse and may cause a vein to be mistaken for an artery.

56. A: Handwritten patient ID labels are often used instead of preprinted labels for blood bank testing because of the serious risks of a transfusion reaction if a patient gets the wrong blood type because a specimen is mislabeled. In order to handwrite a label correctly, the phlebotomist must verify the patient's name, date of birth, and other important information. Errors can occur at any point in collection, processing, and administration.

57. B: Because of the danger posed by sparks in the healthcare environment, the initial response to finding a frayed cord on a piece of equipment should be to unplug the equipment and then follow procedures for reporting that the equipment needs repair, usually to a direct supervisor or to the repair service. If the equipment is covered by a service agreement, the service provider must be notified as well. OSHA regulations regarding electrical safety require that any repair of electrical cords or equipment be performed by qualified and authorized individuals.

58. D: When using a bariatric blood pressure cuff instead of a tourniquet for an obese patient, the blood pressure cuff should be inflated to just below the patient's diastolic pressure. The phlebotomist should begin by measuring the patient's blood pressure and then adjusting the pressure. The cuff should not be so tight that it is painful for the patient. Whereas most tourniquets are approximately 18 inches in length, bariatric tourniquets are available in longer lengths.

59. C: The active safety device on a double-pointed needle is generally activated by pushing the lever forward with the thumb before the needle is removed from the vein so that the safety mechanism slides forward to cover the needle as it is withdrawn. Sharps safety requirements are mandated by OSHA to prevent needlestick injuries and potential exposure of healthcare workers to bloodborne pathogens. Different types of safety devices are available, some of which are activated after the needle is withdrawn.

60. C: Newborn screening should be carried out after the first 24 hours of life. If a neonate is discharged from the hospital prior to 24 hours and tested before discharge, the parent(s) should be advised to have the child retested because some tests are not accurate prior to the first 24 hours. The test is usually carried out with a capillary specimen from a heelstick. Tests included in newborn screening may vary somewhat from one state to another, but typically include tests for metabolic disorders, hormone disorders, hemoglobin disorders, and other rare conditions.

61. C: If a vein collapses during a blood draw, the phlebotomist should apply gentle pressure on the vein above the venipuncture site with a flat index finger so that the vein fills with blood for a couple of seconds and then release, allowing the blood to continue to flow. Veins are most likely to collapse if blood was withdrawn too forcefully or if veins are small and fragile, such as may occur with older adults.

62. B: Whole-blood samples for an activated partial thromboplastin time (aPTT) can remain at room temperature if they will be sent to the lab and tested within a few hours. The exact amount of time that samples can remain at room temperature varies by laboratory. Generally, samples over 4 hours old must be centrifuged and the plasma frozen immediately after transfer into a new tube. This time is reduced (often to 1 hour) if the patient is on heparin therapy. Normal values vary by lab equipment and even test reagent, but are usually around 30–40 seconds. The aPTT is used to monitor the effectiveness of heparin therapy.

63. C: If drawing blood from a metacarpal vein, the tourniquet should be placed 3–4 inches above the wrist bone. Generally, regardless of the venipuncture site, the tourniquet should be placed 3–4 inches above the site. If the tourniquet is too close to the venipuncture site, it may result in a collapsed vessel. If it is too far away from the site, it may be ineffective in dilating the vein. The tourniquet should be applied firmly but not so tightly that it restricts arterial flow (as evidenced by blanching below the tourniquet).

64. C: Hiatal hernia is a condition marked by protrusion of the stomach through a weak area of the diaphragm. Gastritis is an acute or chronic inflammation of the stomach lining. Peptic ulcer is erosion of the stomach lining. Gastroesophageal reflux disease (GERD) is a relaxation of the lower esophageal sphincter muscle, which allows the contents of the stomach to move up the esophagus.

65. B: If a patient is chewing gum while the phlebotomist prepares to draw blood for a CBC, the patient should be asked to remove the gum before the procedure begins. Patients should not have food, gum, or anything else (including a thermometer) in their mouths during a venipuncture because, if the patient experiences pain, they may suddenly inhale, which increases the risk of aspiration; the patient may also bite down or open the mouth in response, which may result in damage to anything held in the mouth.

66. B: If, after leaving a patient's room, the phlebotomist is asked by the patient's brother what tests the patient is having, the phlebotomist should provide no information. Under the federal Health Insurance Portability and Accountability Act (HIPAA), healthcare providers are prohibited from violating an individual's privacy by providing any information about the patient without the explicit permission of the patient. The exception is if the patient is a minor and information is provided to a parent or legal guardian, or if the person asking for information has power of attorney for healthcare for the patient.

67. D: Petechiae, or small red spots that appear on the patient's skin when the tourniquet is applied, are usually caused by capillary wall defects or platelet abnormalities and are indicative of heavy bleeding at the venipuncture site; however, they do not trigger the formation of hematomas. Using veins that are too small or fragile for the size of the needle, applying inadequate pressure to the venipuncture site after the needle is removed, and allowing the needle to penetrate all the way through the vein may lead to hematoma formation.

68. B: PEP (postexposure prophylaxis) is available for exposure to HIV and HBV. However, no PEP is available for HCV (hepatitis C virus), although the CDC does provide a plan for management. If a phlebotomist has a needlestick injury, he or she should immediately wash the area with soap and water, then notify a supervisor and seek medical care in the emergency department or from an appropriate healthcare provider. PEP may not be required in all cases.

69. A: Labeling a tube after collection of a blood sample should be done immediately after completing the venipuncture and while still in the patient's presence per CLSI guidelines. This ensures that the tubes are not confused with those of other patients and mislabeled. Most hospitals provide preprinted labels. If not, a label should be filled out with the patient's first and last name, identification number, date, and time, as well as the phlebotomist's initials. Unlabeled collection tubes should never be taken into the laboratory.

70. B: Following venipuncture with excessive bleeding, a saturated bloodstained gauze should be placed in a hazardous waste container, which should be clearly marked as such. Bloodstained gauze can be deposited in an open trash container, such as a bedside wastebasket, if the blood is dry or the gauze is not saturated. It should never be placed in a sharps container, which should be reserved for needles and other sharps and attached equipment only. Placing gauze in the sharps container may prevent needles from falling to the bottom of the container.

71. A: The aPTT (activated partial thromboplastin time) is most often used to monitor unfractionated heparin therapy. Initially, the test is repeated every 6 hours until the therapeutic range is achieved. The same procedure is followed if the heparin dosage is changed. Once stabilized, the aPTT is usually checked once daily, preferably at the same time each day because some diurnal variation may occur. If the patient is receiving heparin by IV infusion, the blood specimen should be drawn from the opposite arm to avoid heparin contamination of the specimen.

72. B: If an antecubital vein cannot be found on either arm, a capillary puncture may be considered, provided the test can be performed on capillary blood. Veins on the underside of the wrist should not be used because of the high risk of nerve injury. Manipulating the site may change blood composition, which may interfere with test results. Tendons are tough, fibrous connective tissues that are very slow to heal if ruptured and so should not be punctured; furthermore, the blood vessels within tendons are not sufficient for venipuncture.

73. B: When taking calls, the phlebotomist should not wait until the first call is finished before taking another call; ask the first caller for permission to be put on hold, then answer the second call. When the second call is completed, return to the first call. An individual's "personal space," or comfort zone, is based on culture and should be respected. Sign language may be used for hearing-impaired patients who understand sign language. Medical interpreters are extremely helpful in communicating accurately with non-English-speaking patents.

74. C: Medical facilities must review the availability of safer medical devices on an annual basis at the least. OSHA requires that facilities provide safe medical equipment and devices; however, OSHA does not provide information about lists of equipment, so the facility must do a product review to determine when and if safer medical devices have become available. If there is no available device that provides safer options, then medical devices that may expose the healthcare worker to blood or other potentially infectious materials may be utilized with appropriate PPE.

75. D: If blood must be drawn from a 3-year-old, the phlebotomist should explain the procedure to the child, using language and terms that are age-appropriate and taking time to speak with the child before touching him or her because children of this age are often fearful of strangers and pain. When possible, the parent should assist, such as by utilizing a hug hold during the procedure or distracting the child. The phlebotomist should use a soothing tone of voice, praising the child during the venipuncture.

76. B: If, when the phlebotomist is performing a venipuncture in the antecubital space, the patient grabs the arm and complains of severe, shock-like shooting pain, the initial response should be to remove the needle and apply pressure, as these symptoms indicate that the needle has hit a nerve. Continuing the procedure increases the risk of permanent or long-term damage to the nerve; even with prompt removal of the needle, pain may persist for extended periods. Protocol should be followed in reporting and documenting the incident.

77. A: Standard blood specimens do not require chilling for transport and should be transported in a biohazard bag at room temperature. Only specific specimens, such as those to be tested for lactate, require chilling immediately upon collection and during transport; this is indicated in the lab order. The bag should be labeled clearly as a biohazard bag due to its contents containing bodily fluids.

78. D: Blood should not be drawn from an outpatient who is standing or seated on a high or backless stool because of the possibility of fainting. Outpatients should be seated on a special blood-drawing chair or on a chair with armrests; however, if the patient has a tendency to faint, he or she may be seated in a reclining chair or lying down.

79. C: At room temperature, EDTA specimens for erythrocyte sedimentation rate (ESR) must be tested within 4 hours; refrigerated specimens must be tested within 12 hours. The ESR is used to diagnose acute infection or inflammatory processes in disease. The test is typically performed on whole blood collected in a lavender/purple EDTA tube. The test determines how quickly RBCs (erythrocytes) settle to the bottom of the specimen tube. Inflammation or infection tends to speed this process.

80. C: In a hospital environment, infection is most commonly spread by contaminated hands, often those of healthcare workers who carry microorganisms from one patient to another when they fail to carry out adequate handwashing. The hands should be washed both before and after contact with patients, and wearing gloves does not preclude the need for handwashing. Hand cleansing may be done with soap and running water (always needed if residue is present on the hands) or alcohol-based hand rub.

81. C: A collapsed vein may result from the vacuum draw of the tube, pressure from pulling on the syringe, or if the tourniquet is too tight or too close to the venipuncture site. Frequent venipunctures, whether to draw blood or inject medications, can also cause veins to collapse. Stoppage of blood flow when the tourniquet is removed may simply indicate that the needle is not positioned properly; slightly adjusting the needle usually reestablishes blood flow.

82. D: Hydrocephalus is an increased volume of cerebrospinal fluid in the brain at birth and is characterized by an enlargement of the infant's head. Headache, stiff neck, and fever are symptoms of meningitis, or an inflammation of the meninges of the brain. A shuffling gait, muscular rigidity, and tremor are characteristic of Parkinson's disease. Nerve pain is characteristic of neuralgia.

83. D: The blood specimen for the lactic acid test must be immediately chilled because if it remains warm, metabolic processes continue, and this can alter test results. Other tests for which specimens must be chilled include gastrin, ammonia, parathyroid hormone, pH and blood gases, and catecholamines. The tube with the specimen should be placed in crushed ice or a mixture of crushed ice and water, but large ice cubes should not be used as the water temperature may not be stable.

84. D: Specimens for cholesterol testing require centrifugation. Tests that are carried out on whole blood, such as CBC, hemoglobin A1c, whole blood lead analysis, and cyclosporine do not require centrifugation; however, if they are accidentally centrifuged, it may be possible to carry out testing on some specimens after the specimens are examined by a technician. Collection tubes with whole blood specimens are usually placed in a device that gently rocks the tubes while awaiting examination.

85. C: Negligence is defined as the failure to act, resulting in injury or harm to the patient, and does not require intent to harm. Invasion of privacy is a tort involving use of a patient's name for commercial gain, intrusion into the patient's private life, or disclosure of private information. Abandonment is the premature termination of a professional relationship with a patient without notice or patient consent.

86. C: Protective isolation, or reverse isolation, may be required for patients who are highly susceptible to infection, such as burn patients, patients with AIDS, or chemotherapy patients with a low neutrophil count. Protective isolation is usually not required for infants.

87. A: Standard precautions must be used with all patients in all settings in order to protect both the patient and the phlebotomist or other healthcare providers. Standard precautions include using proper hand hygiene (soap and water or alcohol-based rub), using PPE (personal protective

216

equipment) as indicated, following safe injection practices, carrying out safe handling of equipment and environmental surfaces in the patient's environment, and using correct cough hygiene in order to prevent the spread of infection.

88. D: ESR (erythrocyte sedimentation rate), which assesses inflammation, and BUN (blood urea nitrogen), which assesses kidney function, are not usually part of the workup for DIC (disseminated intravascular coagulation). BUN may be ordered later if organ failure is a concern. Tests associated with testing for DIC include Hgb (hemoglobin), Hct (hematocrit), PT (prothrombin time), aPTT (activated partial thromboplastin time), TT (thrombin time), D-dimer, and fibrinogen. DIC is a clotting disorder that causes small clots to block vessels, reducing the number of circulating platelets and causing excessive bleeding.

89. C: In this situation, CLSI guidelines recommend inflating the blood pressure (BP) cuff to slightly below the individual's diastolic BP. Previously, guidelines were to use a pressure of 40 mmHg, but this did not account for patient-specific considerations, in which case that pressure may be excessive (in smaller individuals or individuals with low BP), or insufficient (in individuals that are obese or hypertensive). Once the cuff is inflated, the patient should be asked to gently open and close a fist one or two times, but should never be asked to vigorously pump the fist; even doing so for a short period of time may change the values of some lab results. When using a tourniquet, it is better to avoid all fist pumping.

90. D: When drawing blood from a patient with moderate to advanced dementia, it is most important to ask for assistance because patients with dementia are unreliable in their responses, so a patient who seems very placid may react violently to discomfort because of their inability to comprehend. The phlebotomist should speak soothingly to the patient, explaining for a moment or two before beginning the procedure. The assistant should gently immobilize the venipuncture site to prevent the patient from jerking away during the procedure.

91. D: All varieties of tests for bilirubin—total serum, amniotic fluid, direct, serum, and neonatal—require that the specimen be protected from light. Amber-colored tubes are usually used for specimens that must be protected from light; if these tubes are not available, a clear tube may be used and immediately wrapped in aluminum foil to block light. Other tests that require light protection include those for vitamins C, A, E, B1, B2, and B6, as well as tests for porphyrins and beta-carotene.

92. D: In the hug hold, the parent (or caregiver) sits and holds the toddler, who is facing the parent and enclosed in the parent's arms, with one of the toddler's arms covered by the parent's arm. This secures the toddler physically and also helps the toddler to feel secure and less frightened. The supine position should be avoided with small children, as it leaves them the most exposed, increasing the child's fear. If placed in the side-lying position, the child may instinctively curl into the fetal position.

93. B: The reservoir host is a person, animal, plant, or other organism or substance that acts as the source of transmission of a pathogen. The susceptible host is the person capable of being infected with a pathogen. Direct contact is the direct physical transfer of pathogens from a reservoir to a susceptible host. The chain of infection is the order in which pathogens are transmitted.

94. D: The vaccination that is not routinely recommended for phlebotomists is HZV (herpes zoster virus). However, because phlebotomists come into close contact with blood, they should have the HBV (hepatitis B virus) series. MMR (measles, mumps, and rubella) vaccination is especially important because so many parents opt to not vaccinate their children, increasing risks of infection.

Yearly influenza vaccinations are usually required for those working with the public. The varicella (chickenpox) vaccination is also usually recommended for phlebotomists.

95. C: The phlebotomist should always verify a patient's ID, even if he or she has been identified by the receptionist or has responded when his or her name has been called. Some outpatients may have been issued an ID card by the clinic; however, outpatients should still be asked to confirm their name and date of birth.

96. D: Bandages are usually avoided in children younger than 2 years because they pose a choking hazard. Young children are usually very flexible and may remove a bandage, such as one applied to a heelstick site, and then place the bandage in their mouth. Instead of a bandage, the phlebotomist should maintain pressure on a puncture or venipuncture site and elevate the extremity for 2–3 minutes, then check to make sure that all bleeding has stopped.

97. B: The accession number, time of test, patient's name and date of birth, and the phlebotomist's initials are required information on specimen tube labels. The physician's signature is required on requisition forms.

98. D: If the laboratory protocol calls for the use of chlorhexidine solution for skin antisepsis for skin puncture or venipuncture, the antiseptic should not be used on infants younger than 2 months. Chlorhexidine solutions are effective against both gram-negative and gram-positive organisms as well as yeasts. Chlorhexidine is often combined with isopropyl alcohol (2% chlorhexidine with 70% isopropyl alcohol) for one-step skin antisepsis. In other cases, skin prep consists of first using 70% isopropyl alcohol and then 2% tincture of iodine.

99. B: The activated clotting time (ACT) test is used to monitor the effectiveness of heparin and to adjust the dose as needed. Partial pressure of oxygen (pO_2) is an arterial blood gas value. Ionized calcium is an electrolyte. Glucose levels are measured by the 2-hour postprandial (PP) test.

100. B: When performing venipuncture on a patient with extensive burns, the phlebotomist should avoid burned areas because of impaired circulation and trauma. If burns are extensive and cover both arms, then alternate sites, such as an ankle, may need to be used. In some cases, skin puncture may allow for collection of small amounts of blood. If a central venous line is in place, blood can be drawn from that access device by appropriate healthcare personnel.

101. B: Partial pressure of oxygen, or pO_2, is used to measure oxygen levels in the blood; decreased oxygen levels increase the respiration rate, and increasing the oxygen level will reduce the respiratory rate. Partial pressure of carbon dioxide, or pCO_2, is used to measure carbon dioxide levels in the blood; increased CO_2 levels in the blood increase the respiration rate and decreasing the pCO_2 will decrease the respiratory rate. HCO_3 measures the amount of bicarbonate in the blood and is used to evaluate the bicarbonate system in the kidneys. The acidity or alkalinity of the blood is measured with the pH.

102. A: If plasma is needed for a chemistry test, the blood may be collected in a tube containing lithium heparin or sodium heparin. Collection tubes that contain lithium heparin and gel for plasma separation are light green- or gray-capped require 8 inversions after collection. Collection tubes that contain sodium heparin or lithium heparin (without gel) are dark green-capped also require 8 inversions after collection.

103. C: The prothrombin time (PT) test may be used in conjunction with partial thromboplastin time (PTT) to assess a patient's total clotting abnormalities. Activated coagulation time (ACT) is used to monitor heparin therapy. Activated partial thromboplastin time (aPTT) is another blood clotting test. PP is postprandial testing, which refers to a test given after a meal.

104. D: Drugs and alcohol testing can be run on blood urine, and hair, but only one or two of these may be required for a specific test. Drug and alcohol testing generally requires patient consent; however, state laws may permit such testing without consent in some situations, such as the patient facing felony drug charges. A proctor may be required to be present to verify that the specimen was obtained from the correct individual. Glass tubes are preferred for blood alcohol specimens because of the porous nature of plastic tubes, but plastic tubes can be used for many drug tests and alcohol tests that will be performed right away. A split sample may be required for confirmation or parallel testing.

105. D: Personal protective equipment (PPE) such as gloves, mask, and gown is required when entering the room of a patient under drainage/secretion isolation, such as those with skin infections; AFB isolation, such as those with tuberculosis; or enteric isolation, such as those with intestinal infections that may be transmitted through ingestion. PPE is not required for entering the room of a patient with HIV.

106. A: If a patient states he has severe needle phobia (trypanophobia), the phlebotomist should have the patient lie flat for the venipuncture because the patient may faint if sitting upright. The phlebotomist should remain supportive but should not assure the patient that the venipuncture will not hurt (because it may) or that it will be fast (because it may not). Phobias are irrational fears and are often unrelated to actual pain. The phlebotomist should ascertain from the patient what may provide the most support, such as a spouse holding the patient's hand or listening to music.

107. D: A phlebotomist who wears contact lenses should wear protective goggles in the laboratory. While contact lenses may provide barrier protection in some cases of eye splashes, they can also pose problems. Some chemicals can penetrate soft lenses, with the lens then holding the substance in place against the cornea. Hard lenses can entrap foreign substances and material beneath them, resulting in abrasion of or other damage to the cornea. OSHA (Occupational Safety and Health Administration) allows the use of contact lenses with respirators.

108. C: B-type natriuretic peptide (BNP) blood concentrations are measured to detect congestive heart failure. The purified protein derivative (PPD) skin test is used to test for tuberculosis. Histoplasma and coccidioidal skin tests are used to test for the fungal infections histoplasmosis and coccidioidomycosis, respectively.

109. D: The method that may prevent hemoconcentration during a venipuncture is to advise the patient to avoid pumping their fist. The patient should also be told to open the hand when blood begins to flow, and the tourniquet should be released within 1 minute. Massaging the vein excessively or squeezing the tissue prior to venipuncture may force some of the fluid in the plasma into capillaries and surrounding tissue, also resulting in hemoconcentration.

110. C: An increased eosinophil count often indicates an allergic reaction, as eosinophils help to moderate these reactions. Eosinophils also increase in the presence of parasites as they try to defend the body. Eosinophils typically comprise only 1–3% of the total number of WBCs. Eosinophil count may also increase with some diseases, including cancer (such as Hodgkin and non-Hodgkin lymphomas), pernicious anemia, rheumatoid arthritis, and tuberculosis. Eosinophil count may decrease with aplastic anemia, eclampsia, infections (associated with left shift), and stress.

111. A: The medial or lateral plantar surface of the heel is the preferred site for capillary puncture in infants. The earlobe or arch or other areas of the foot should not be used for puncture. The posterior curvature of the heel should not be used, as the bone may be only 1 mm deep in this area.

112. D: Cryoglobulin, cryofibrinogen, and cold agglutinin specimens must be kept at or near body temperature. Lactic acid, ammonia, and glucagon specimens require chilling.

113. A: A patent hospitalized for chemotherapy for renal (kidney) cancer would most likely be treated in the oncology (cancer) department. The oncology department specializes in administration of chemotherapy, radiation, and other therapies for the treatment of all types of cancers. Hematology is the specialty that diagnoses and treats diseases of the blood. Endocrinology is the specialty related to endocrine glands and hormones. Cardiology is the branch of medicine that focuses on the heart.

114. D: Blood glucose levels are usually lowest in the morning. Iron, insulin, and potassium levels are usually highest in the morning.

115. B: To prevent hemoconcentration during venipuncture, the phlebotomist should ask the patient to release his or her fist when blood begins to flow; fist-pumping may increase blood potassium levels and should not be encouraged. Excessively massaging the site or probing or redirecting the needle multiple times may result in hemoconcentration.

116. D: The type of microorganism that is usually the causative agent in sepsis is bacteria that have entered the bloodstream, often from a local infection such as a urinary tract infection or pneumonia. Sepsis may also occur after elective surgery or a minor injury. Sepsis is characterized by high fever, chills, tachycardia (rapid heart rate), tachypnea (rapid breathing), nausea and vomiting, elevated WBC count, and positive blood culture. Treatment for sepsis includes intravenous antibiotics.

117. C: When collecting a blood specimen from a 2-month-old infant, the primary interactions will be between the phlebotomist and the parent, who may need reassurance. The phlebotomist should explain the procedure to the parent, using a calm tone of voice, and encourage the parent to hold or maintain other physical contact with the infant during the procedure, which is usually a heelstick. The minimum amount of blood necessary to conduct the tests should be collected.

118. D: According to the order of draw, the blood culture bottle should be filled first to ensure that the specimen remains sterile with no contamination. This is followed by the light-blue–capped tube (which contains a citrate additive). Next is the red and black-capped tube (which may or may not contain a clot activator or gel plasma separator) and last the green-capped tube (which contains heparin).

119. D: The white blood cell type that is most likely to increase in number in response to bacterial infection is the neutrophil. Neutrophils are granulocytes and are characterized by fine granules that appear light purple with combined acid and base stains. These cells are also called polymorphonuclear leukocytes (PMNs). Sometimes, older neutrophils are referred to as "segs" because older neutrophils have multi-lobed (segmented) nuclei connected by thin strands of chromatin. Younger neutrophils are called "bands" because their nuclei are C-shaped.

120. D: Laboratory requisition forms may be transmitted to the laboratory via courier, pneumatic tube system, or in the case of computerized forms, e-mail. Verbal laboratory requests may only be given in the outpatient or emergency setting, and must be documented on a laboratory requisition form as soon as possible.

How to Overcome Test Anxiety

Just the thought of taking a test is enough to make most people a little nervous. A test is an important event that can have a long-term impact on your future, so it's important to take it seriously and it's natural to feel anxious about performing well. But just because anxiety is normal, that doesn't mean that it's helpful in test taking, or that you should simply accept it as part of your life. Anxiety can have a variety of effects. These effects can be mild, like making you feel slightly nervous, or severe, like blocking your ability to focus or remember even a simple detail.

If you experience test anxiety—whether severe or mild—it's important to know how to beat it. To discover this, first you need to understand what causes test anxiety.

Causes of Test Anxiety

While we often think of anxiety as an uncontrollable emotional state, it can actually be caused by simple, practical things. One of the most common causes of test anxiety is that a person does not feel adequately prepared for their test. This feeling can be the result of many different issues such as poor study habits or lack of organization, but the most common culprit is time management. Starting to study too late, failing to organize your study time to cover all of the material, or being distracted while you study will mean that you're not well prepared for the test. This may lead to cramming the night before, which will cause you to be physically and mentally exhausted for the test. Poor time management also contributes to feelings of stress, fear, and hopelessness as you realize you are not well prepared but don't know what to do about it.

Other times, test anxiety is not related to your preparation for the test but comes from unresolved fear. This may be a past failure on a test, or poor performance on tests in general. It may come from comparing yourself to others who seem to be performing better or from the stress of living up to expectations. Anxiety may be driven by fears of the future—how failure on this test would affect your educational and career goals. These fears are often completely irrational, but they can still negatively impact your test performance.

Elements of Test Anxiety

As mentioned earlier, test anxiety is considered to be an emotional state, but it has physical and mental components as well. Sometimes you may not even realize that you are suffering from test anxiety until you notice the physical symptoms. These can include trembling hands, rapid heartbeat, sweating, nausea, and tense muscles. Extreme anxiety may lead to fainting or vomiting. Obviously, any of these symptoms can have a negative impact on testing. It is important to recognize them as soon as they begin to occur so that you can address the problem before it damages your performance.

The mental components of test anxiety include trouble focusing and inability to remember learned information. During a test, your mind is on high alert, which can help you recall information and stay focused for an extended period of time. However, anxiety interferes with your mind's natural processes, causing you to blank out, even on the questions you know well. The strain of testing during anxiety makes it difficult to stay focused, especially on a test that may take several hours. Extreme anxiety can take a huge mental toll, making it difficult not only to recall test information but even to understand the test questions or pull your thoughts together.

221

Effects of Test Anxiety

Test anxiety is like a disease—if left untreated, it will get progressively worse. Anxiety leads to poor performance, and this reinforces the feelings of fear and failure, which in turn lead to poor performances on subsequent tests. It can grow from a mild nervousness to a crippling condition. If allowed to progress, test anxiety can have a big impact on your schooling, and consequently on your future.

Test anxiety can spread to other parts of your life. Anxiety on tests can become anxiety in any stressful situation, and blanking on a test can turn into panicking in a job situation. But fortunately, you don't have to let anxiety rule your testing and determine your grades. There are a number of relatively simple steps you can take to move past anxiety and function normally on a test and in the rest of life.

Physical Steps for Beating Test Anxiety

While test anxiety is a serious problem, the good news is that it can be overcome. It doesn't have to control your ability to think and remember information. While it may take time, you can begin taking steps today to beat anxiety.

Just as your first hint that you may be struggling with anxiety comes from the physical symptoms, the first step to treating it is also physical. Rest is crucial for having a clear, strong mind. If you are tired, it is much easier to give in to anxiety. But if you establish good sleep habits, your body and mind will be ready to perform optimally, without the strain of exhaustion. Additionally, sleeping well helps you to retain information better, so you're more likely to recall the answers when you see the test questions.

Getting good sleep means more than going to bed on time. It's important to allow your brain time to relax. Take study breaks from time to time so it doesn't get overworked, and don't study right before bed. Take time to rest your mind before trying to rest your body, or you may find it difficult to fall asleep.

Along with sleep, other aspects of physical health are important in preparing for a test. Good nutrition is vital for good brain function. Sugary foods and drinks may give a burst of energy but this burst is followed by a crash, both physically and emotionally. Instead, fuel your body with protein and vitamin-rich foods.

Also, drink plenty of water. Dehydration can lead to headaches and exhaustion, especially if your brain is already under stress from the rigors of the test. Particularly if your test is a long one, drink water during the breaks. And if possible, take an energy-boosting snack to eat between sections.

Along with sleep and diet, a third important part of physical health is exercise. Maintaining a steady workout schedule is helpful, but even taking 5-minute study breaks to walk can help get your blood pumping faster and clear your head. Exercise also releases endorphins, which contribute to a positive feeling and can help combat test anxiety.

When you nurture your physical health, you are also contributing to your mental health. If your body is healthy, your mind is much more likely to be healthy as well. So take time to rest, nourish your body with healthy food and water, and get moving as much as possible. Taking these physical steps will make you stronger and more able to take the mental steps necessary to overcome test anxiety.

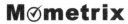

Mental Steps for Beating Test Anxiety

Working on the mental side of test anxiety can be more challenging, but as with the physical side, there are clear steps you can take to overcome it. As mentioned earlier, test anxiety often stems from lack of preparation, so the obvious solution is to prepare for the test. Effective studying may be the most important weapon you have for beating test anxiety, but you can and should employ several other mental tools to combat fear.

First, boost your confidence by reminding yourself of past success—tests or projects that you aced. If you're putting as much effort into preparing for this test as you did for those, there's no reason you should expect to fail here. Work hard to prepare; then trust your preparation.

Second, surround yourself with encouraging people. It can be helpful to find a study group, but be sure that the people you're around will encourage a positive attitude. If you spend time with others who are anxious or cynical, this will only contribute to your own anxiety. Look for others who are motivated to study hard from a desire to succeed, not from a fear of failure.

Third, reward yourself. A test is physically and mentally tiring, even without anxiety, and it can be helpful to have something to look forward to. Plan an activity following the test, regardless of the outcome, such as going to a movie or getting ice cream.

When you are taking the test, if you find yourself beginning to feel anxious, remind yourself that you know the material. Visualize successfully completing the test. Then take a few deep, relaxing breaths and return to it. Work through the questions carefully but with confidence, knowing that you are capable of succeeding.

Developing a healthy mental approach to test taking will also aid in other areas of life. Test anxiety affects more than just the actual test—it can be damaging to your mental health and even contribute to depression. It's important to beat test anxiety before it becomes a problem for more than testing.

Study Strategy

Being prepared for the test is necessary to combat anxiety, but what does being prepared look like? You may study for hours on end and still not feel prepared. What you need is a strategy for test prep. The next few pages outline our recommended steps to help you plan out and conquer the challenge of preparation.

STEP 1: SCOPE OUT THE TEST

Learn everything you can about the format (multiple choice, essay, etc.) and what will be on the test. Gather any study materials, course outlines, or sample exams that may be available. Not only will this help you to prepare, but knowing what to expect can help to alleviate test anxiety.

STEP 2: MAP OUT THE MATERIAL

Look through the textbook or study guide and make note of how many chapters or sections it has. Then divide these over the time you have. For example, if a book has 15 chapters and you have five days to study, you need to cover three chapters each day. Even better, if you have the time, leave an extra day at the end for overall review after you have gone through the material in depth.

If time is limited, you may need to prioritize the material. Look through it and make note of which sections you think you already have a good grasp on, and which need review. While you are studying, skim quickly through the familiar sections and take more time on the challenging parts.

Write out your plan so you don't get lost as you go. Having a written plan also helps you feel more in control of the study, so anxiety is less likely to arise from feeling overwhelmed at the amount to cover.

STEP 3: GATHER YOUR TOOLS

Decide what study method works best for you. Do you prefer to highlight in the book as you study and then go back over the highlighted portions? Or do you type out notes of the important information? Or is it helpful to make flashcards that you can carry with you? Assemble the pens, index cards, highlighters, post-it notes, and any other materials you may need so you won't be distracted by getting up to find things while you study.

If you're having a hard time retaining the information or organizing your notes, experiment with different methods. For example, try color-coding by subject with colored pens, highlighters, or post-it notes. If you learn better by hearing, try recording yourself reading your notes so you can listen while in the car, working out, or simply sitting at your desk. Ask a friend to quiz you from your flashcards, or try teaching someone the material to solidify it in your mind.

STEP 4: CREATE YOUR ENVIRONMENT

It's important to avoid distractions while you study. This includes both the obvious distractions like visitors and the subtle distractions like an uncomfortable chair (or a too-comfortable couch that makes you want to fall asleep). Set up the best study environment possible: good lighting and a comfortable work area. If background music helps you focus, you may want to turn it on, but otherwise keep the room quiet. If you are using a computer to take notes, be sure you don't have any other windows open, especially applications like social media, games, or anything else that could distract you. Silence your phone and turn off notifications. Be sure to keep water close by so you stay hydrated while you study (but avoid unhealthy drinks and snacks).

Also, take into account the best time of day to study. Are you freshest first thing in the morning? Try to set aside some time then to work through the material. Is your mind clearer in the afternoon or evening? Schedule your study session then. Another method is to study at the same time of day that you will take the test, so that your brain gets used to working on the material at that time and will be ready to focus at test time.

STEP 5: STUDY!

Once you have done all the study preparation, it's time to settle into the actual studying. Sit down, take a few moments to settle your mind so you can focus, and begin to follow your study plan. Don't give in to distractions or let yourself procrastinate. This is your time to prepare so you'll be ready to fearlessly approach the test. Make the most of the time and stay focused.

Of course, you don't want to burn out. If you study too long you may find that you're not retaining the information very well. Take regular study breaks. For example, taking five minutes out of every hour to walk briskly, breathing deeply and swinging your arms, can help your mind stay fresh.

As you get to the end of each chapter or section, it's a good idea to do a quick review. Remind yourself of what you learned and work on any difficult parts. When you feel that you've mastered the material, move on to the next part. At the end of your study session, briefly skim through your notes again.

But while review is helpful, cramming last minute is NOT. If at all possible, work ahead so that you won't need to fit all your study into the last day. Cramming overloads your brain with more information than it can process and retain, and your tired mind may struggle to recall even previously learned information when it is overwhelmed with last-minute study. Also, the urgent nature of cramming and the stress placed on your brain contribute to anxiety. You'll be more likely to go to the test feeling unprepared and having trouble thinking clearly.

So don't cram, and don't stay up late before the test, even just to review your notes at a leisurely pace. Your brain needs rest more than it needs to go over the information again. In fact, plan to finish your studies by noon or early afternoon the day before the test. Give your brain the rest of the day to relax or focus on other things, and get a good night's sleep. Then you will be fresh for the test and better able to recall what you've studied.

Step 6: Take a Practice Test

Many courses offer sample tests, either online or in the study materials. This is an excellent resource to check whether you have mastered the material, as well as to prepare for the test format and environment.

Check the test format ahead of time: the number of questions, the type (multiple choice, free response, etc.), and the time limit. Then create a plan for working through them. For example, if you have 30 minutes to take a 60-question test, your limit is 30 seconds per question. Spend less time on the questions you know well so that you can take more time on the difficult ones.

If you have time to take several practice tests, take the first one open book, with no time limit. Work through the questions at your own pace and make sure you fully understand them. Gradually work up to taking a test under test conditions: sit at a desk with all study materials put away and set a timer. Pace yourself to make sure you finish the test with time to spare and go back to check your answers if you have time.

After each test, check your answers. On the questions you missed, be sure you understand why you missed them. Did you misread the question (tests can use tricky wording)? Did you forget the information? Or was it something you hadn't learned? Go back and study any shaky areas that the practice tests reveal.

Taking these tests not only helps with your grade, but also aids in combating test anxiety. If you're already used to the test conditions, you're less likely to worry about it, and working through tests until you're scoring well gives you a confidence boost. Go through the practice tests until you feel comfortable, and then you can go into the test knowing that you're ready for it.

Test Tips

On test day, you should be confident, knowing that you've prepared well and are ready to answer the questions. But aside from preparation, there are several test day strategies you can employ to maximize your performance.

First, as stated before, get a good night's sleep the night before the test (and for several nights before that, if possible). Go into the test with a fresh, alert mind rather than staying up late to study.

Try not to change too much about your normal routine on the day of the test. It's important to eat a nutritious breakfast, but if you normally don't eat breakfast at all, consider eating just a protein bar. If you're a coffee drinker, go ahead and have your normal coffee. Just make sure you time it so that the caffeine doesn't wear off right in the middle of your test. Avoid sugary beverages, and drink enough water to stay hydrated but not so much that you need a restroom break 10 minutes into the

225

test. If your test isn't first thing in the morning, consider going for a walk or doing a light workout before the test to get your blood flowing.

Allow yourself enough time to get ready, and leave for the test with plenty of time to spare so you won't have the anxiety of scrambling to arrive in time. Another reason to be early is to select a good seat. It's helpful to sit away from doors and windows, which can be distracting. Find a good seat, get out your supplies, and settle your mind before the test begins.

When the test begins, start by going over the instructions carefully, even if you already know what to expect. Make sure you avoid any careless mistakes by following the directions.

Then begin working through the questions, pacing yourself as you've practiced. If you're not sure on an answer, don't spend too much time on it, and don't let it shake your confidence. Either skip it and come back later, or eliminate as many wrong answers as possible and guess among the remaining ones. Don't dwell on these questions as you continue—put them out of your mind and focus on what lies ahead.

Be sure to read all of the answer choices, even if you're sure the first one is the right answer. Sometimes you'll find a better one if you keep reading. But don't second-guess yourself if you do immediately know the answer. Your gut instinct is usually right. Don't let test anxiety rob you of the information you know.

If you have time at the end of the test (and if the test format allows), go back and review your answers. Be cautious about changing any, since your first instinct tends to be correct, but make sure you didn't misread any of the questions or accidentally mark the wrong answer choice. Look over any you skipped and make an educated guess.

At the end, leave the test feeling confident. You've done your best, so don't waste time worrying about your performance or wishing you could change anything. Instead, celebrate the successful completion of this test. And finally, use this test to learn how to deal with anxiety even better next time.

> **Review Video: Test Anxiety**
> Visit mometrix.com/academy and enter code: 100340

Important Qualification

Not all anxiety is created equal. If your test anxiety is causing major issues in your life beyond the classroom or testing center, or if you are experiencing troubling physical symptoms related to your anxiety, it may be a sign of a serious physiological or psychological condition. If this sounds like your situation, we strongly encourage you to seek professional help.

Additional Bonus Material

Due to our efforts to try to keep this book to a manageable length, we've created a link that will give you access to all of your additional bonus material:

mometrix.com/bonus948/nhaphleb

227